1986

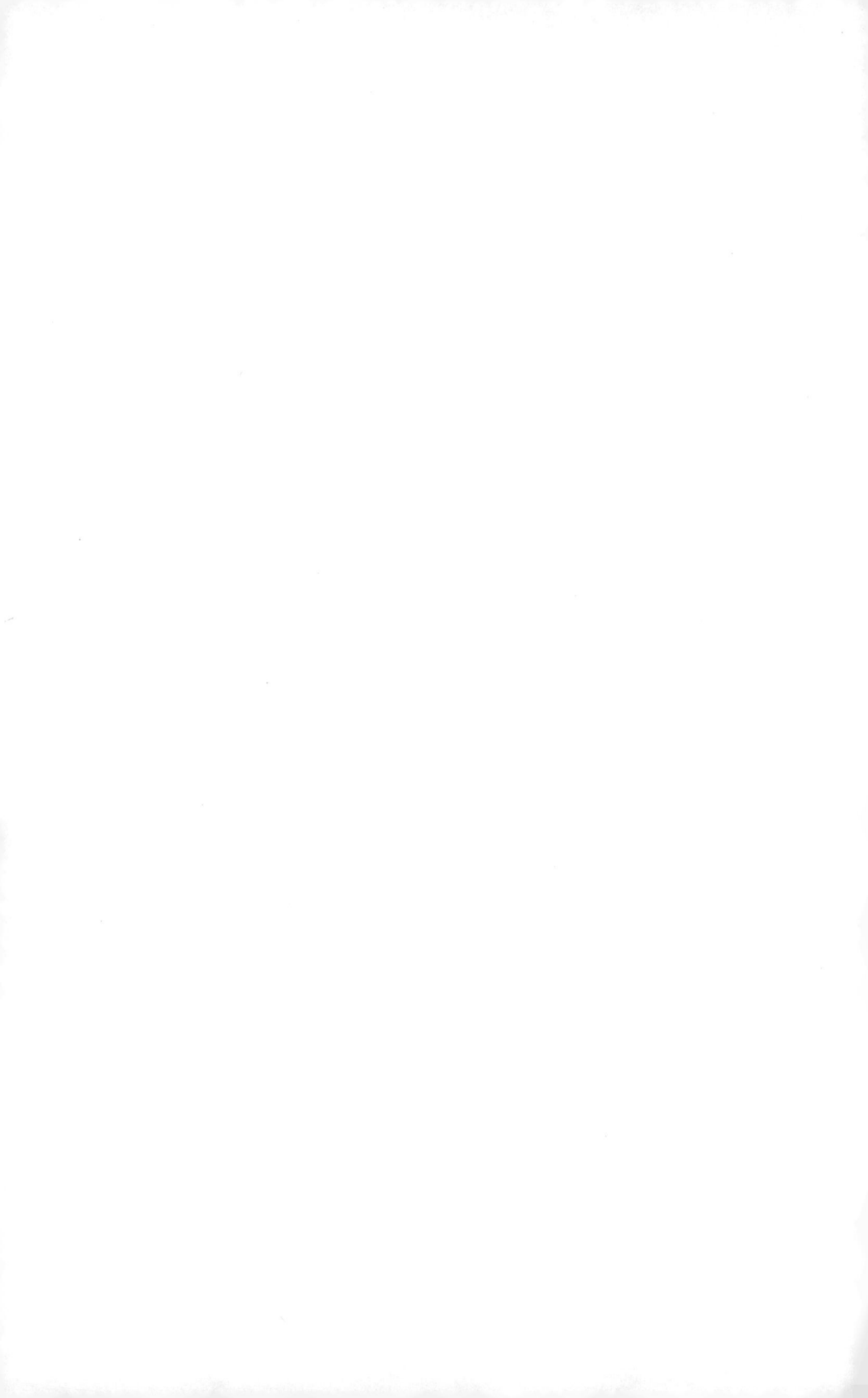

Proteinuria and the Nephrotic Syndrome

Proteinuria and the Nephrotic Syndrome

DONALD E. HRICIK, M.D.
Assistant Professor of Medicine
Case Western Reserve University
Cleveland, Ohio

MICHAEL C. SMITH, M.D.
Associate Professor of Medicine
Chairman, Division of General Medicine
Case Western Reserve University
Cleveland, Ohio

YEAR BOOK MEDICAL PUBLISHERS, INC.
CHICAGO • LONDON

Copyright © 1986 by Year Book Medical Publishers, Inc. All rights reserved. No part of this publication may be reproduced, stored in a retrieval system, or transmitted, in any form or by any means, electronic, mechanical, photocopying, recording, or otherwise, without prior written permission from the publisher. Printed in the United States of America.

0 9 8 7 6 5 4 3 2 1

Library of Congress Cataloging-in-Publication Data

Hricik, Donald E.
  Proteinuria and the nephrotic syndrome.

  Include bibliographies and index.
  1. Nephrotic syndrome. 2. Proteinuria. I. Smith, Michael C. (Michael Charles), 1946–   . II. Title.
  [DNLM: 1. Nephrotic Syndrome. 2. Proteinuria. WJ 343 H873p]
  RC918.N43H75   1986   616.6'1   85-20216
  ISBN 0-8151-4717-1

Sponsoring editor: Richard H. Lampert
Manager, copyediting services: Frances M. Perveiler
Production project manager: Sharon W. Pepping
Proofroom supervisor: Shirley E. Taylor

To Our Families:

Lynne Hricik
Brian, Kevin, Lauren

Kathy Smith
Michael, Brian, Patrick

Preface

THE EXCRETION of excessive urinary protein is a cardinal sign of renal disease and forms the physiologic basis for one of the most dramatic syndromes in clinical nephrology—the nephrotic syndrome. Although nephrologists are frequently consulted to treat patients with the nephrotic syndrome, the initial evaluation and long-term management of patients with proteinuria are more often responsibilities of the primary care physician. All physicians who employ the "routine urinalysis" as a screening procedure in clinical practice must be familiar with the causes, mechanisms, and consequences of proteinuria. As general internists and nephrologists, we have written this book with an emphasis on practical aspects of diagnosis and management of interest to non-nephrologists who treat patients with proteinuria. By devoting a major segment of the book to disorders accompanied by heavy proteinuria, we also offer a review for practicing nephrologists who care for patients with the nephrotic syndrome.

While focusing on glomerular diseases associated with the nephrotic syndrome, we have attempted to consider this syndrome within the context of a broader classification of proteinuric states, including those more commonly encountered in a general practice. For the primary physician, recognition of both qualitative and quantitative patterns of urinary protein excretion is the first step in formulating a diagnostic and therapeutic plan for the proteinuric patient. In Chapter 1, we discuss methods for the detection of urinary protein and provide a classification of proteinuric states as a foundation for the remainder of the book. Mechanisms accounting for enhanced urinary protein excretion in both glomerular and nonglomerular renal diseases are reviewed in Chapter 2.

Chapters 3 through 5 deal exclusively with glomerular diseases accompanied by heavy proteinuria and the nephrotic syndrome. In Chapter 3, we discuss the common consequences and potential life-threatening complications of heavy proteinuria per se. The renal histology, pathophysiology, clinical features, and specific therapy for the nephrotic syndrome resulting from systemic disorders (i.e., *secondary* nephrotic syndrome) are reviewed in detail in Chapter 4. Chapter 5 provides a similar profile for the glomerulopathies underlying the idiopathic (i.e., *primary*) nephrotic syndrome.

No specific therapy is available for many of the disorders associated with the nephrotic syndrome. Moreover, patients with "treatable" glomerular diseases not infrequently become refractory to specific therapy. Thus, the primary physician often is involved in the long-term management of the nephrotic patient long after an initial referral to a renal specialist. In Chapter 6, we discuss the general management of patients with persistent nephrotic syndrome and other disorders associated with lesser degrees of proteinuria. Finally, we provide a series of illustrative cases in Chapter 7 to highlight issues in the diagnosis and management of proteinuric patients.

The compilation of this book, geared both to primary physicians and nephrologists, has been almost as challenging as the day-to-day management of the patients about whom it is written! Our understanding of the mechanisms and consequences of proteinuria has expanded rapidly during the past two decades, but much remains to be learned about the basic causes and treatments of renal diseases accompanied by excessive urinary protein excretion. For many of the disorders discussed herein, uniformly accepted approaches to diagnosis and treatment have not been established. In such cases, we have taken the liberty of outlining our own management policies—but only with the understanding that future research in this important area of nephrology may radically alter our current approach to the diagnosis and treatment of patients with proteinuria.

We would like to express our thanks to Drs. Gretta Jacobs and Steven Emancipator who provided pathologic material for the book. We also acknowledge Diane Kastelnick for assistance with the artwork and Sharon Nash for clerical assistance with the manuscript.

DONALD E. HRICIK, M.D.
MICHAEL C. SMITH, M.D.

Contents

PREFACE vii

1 / Detection and Classification of Proteinuric States 1

    Methods for Detection and Quantitation of Proteinuria 2
    Approach to the "Healthy" Patient With a Positive
    Test for Urine Protein 7
    Classification of Proteinuric States 8
    Appendix 13

2 / Mechanisms of Proteinuria 17

    Protein-Handling by the Normal Kidney 17
    Mechanisms of Proteinuria in Renal Disease 25
    Mechanisms of Proteinuria in Nonglomerular Renal Disease:
        The Role of Intrarenal Hemodynamic Factors 31
    Immunologic Mechanisms of Glomerular Injury 32
    Mechanisms of Functional Proteinuria 39

**3 / The Nephrotic Syndrome: Consequences of Heavy
Proteinuria** 45

    Common Consequences of Heavy Proteinuria 46
    Miscellaneous Consequences of Heavy Proteinuria 54
    Life-Threatening Complications of Heavy Proteinuria 59

**4 / Disorders Associated With Secondary Nephrotic
Syndrome** 69

    Diabetes Mellitus 69
    Systemic Lupus Erythematosus 80
    Amyloidosis 90
    Drugs and Toxins 95
    Malignancy 101

x   *Contents*

    Infectious Diseases 105
    Pregnancy. 109
    Miscellaneous Causes of Nephrotic Syndrome 110

5 / Idiopathic Nephrotic Syndrome 119
    Membranous Glomerulopathy. 119
    Minimal Change Disease. 127
    Focal Glomerular Sclerosis 133
    Membranoproliferative Glomerulonephritis 138
    Miscellaneous Proliferative Lesions 143

6 / Diagnosis and General Management of the
Proteinuric Patient 149
    Assessment and Management of Patients With Intermittent
      or Asymptomatic Proteinuria 150
    Assessment and Management of Patients With Heavy
      Proteinuria and the Nephrotic Syndrome 152
    The Role of Renal Biopsy in Patients With Idiopathic
      Nephrotic Syndrome. 155
    Management of Metabolic Abnormalities Associated
      With the Nephrotic Syndrome. 157
    Management of Other Consequences of Heavy Proteinuria. . . . 165
    Management of Children With the Nephrotic Syndrome. 169

7 / Illustrative Cases 175
    Patient 1. A Woman With Congestive Heart Failure
      and Nephrotic Syndrome. 175
    Patient 2. A Man With Flank Pain and Gross Hematuria 177
    Patient 3. A Child With Frequently Relapsing
      Nephrotic Syndrome. 179
    Patient 4. A College Student With Intermittent
      Proteinuria 181
    Patient 5. A Woman With Rheumatoid Arthritis and Heavy
      Proteinuria 182
    Patient 6. A Young Man With Hodgkin's Disease
      and Nephrotic Syndrome. 184
    Patient 7. A Kidney Transplant Recipient
      With Heavy Proteinuria 185
    Patient 8. An Elderly Woman With Nephrotic Syndrome 186

INDEX **189**

1 Detection and Classification of Proteinuric States

THE UPPER LIMIT OF urinary protein excretion in healthy adults is approximately 150 mg per day. One third of the protein in normal urine consists of albumin; the remaining proteins include a number of globulins, most of which have immunologically identical counterparts in serum. Normal urine also contains small amounts of glycoproteins, presumably secreted by the epithelium of the urinary tract. The major protein in normal urine that has no counterpart in serum is Tamm-Horsfall protein, a large glycoprotein secreted by distal renal tubular cells in amounts of 30 to 60 mg per day.[1] Because the urine of normal healthy subjects contains small amounts of protein, it is the quantity and not the mere presence of urinary protein that defines an abnormal state.

Excretion of *excessive* amounts of urinary protein is characteristic of most renal diseases. Indeed, relatively few disorders cause impairment of renal function without a simultaneous increase in the protein content of urine (Table 1–1). Even among the disorders listed in Table 1–1, absence of proteinuria is more often the exception than the rule, especially when the underlying disorder is associated with long-standing renal insufficiency. It is the possibility of underlying renal disease with the potential for end-stage renal failure that makes the detection of even small amounts of urinary protein a matter of concern for both the patient and the physician. In addition to the concern that proteinuria may be the first sign of renal disease, its discovery may have other serious implications for the patient such as rejection from military service, job disqualification, or denial of life insurance. Thus, a positive test for urine protein always warrants investigation.

Detection of excessive urinary protein does not always indicate underlying renal disease. A reversible increase in urinary protein excre-

TABLE 1-1.—RENAL DISORDERS
IN WHICH PROTEINURIA MAY
BE ABSENT

Interstitial nephritis
Urinary tract infection
Obstructive uropathy
Nephrolithiasis
Polycystic kidney disease
Hypercalcemic
  nephropathy
Hypokalemic
  nephropathy

---

tion occurs in a variety of physiologic and pathologic settings in the absence of renal parenchymal injury. Furthermore, the methods employed as screening tests for proteinuria are subject to false-positive results. There is little doubt about the presence of underlying renal disease in the patient who presents with heavy proteinuria and its clinical counterpart, the nephrotic syndrome. More commonly encountered in clinical practice is the asymptomatic, apparently healthy patient who simply has a positive test for urine protein. In deciding whether such a patient has covert renal disease, functional proteinuria, or a false-positive test, the physician must rely on a careful assessment of the overall clinical picture, including information obtained from a complete medical history, physical examination, and a few simple laboratory tests of renal function. The nature and extent of the diagnostic evaluation of the patient with a positive test for urine protein are further dictated by quantitation of urine protein and by recognition of specific patterns of abnormal protein excretion. In the remainder of the chapter, we review methods employed for the detection and quantitation of urinary protein, consider the approach to the "healthy" patient with a positive test for urine protein, and provide a classification scheme for various proteinuric states based on qualitative and quantitative patterns of proteinuria.

METHODS FOR DETECTION AND QUANTITATION OF PROTEINURIA

Of the tests available for measurement of urinary protein, quantitative analyses in timed urine collections are the most useful in assessing the presence and severity of underlying renal disease and in monitoring therapy, but they are not practical for routine screening purposes. Collection of 24-hour urine specimens is cumbersome and errors in the collection procedure are frequent, especially when specimens are obtained on an outpatient basis. Semiquantitative tests of protein excretion in random urine samples are more appropriate for screening.

Semiquantitative Assays for Proteinuria

Semiquantitative tests involve either protein-induced color changes of an indicator dye on a dipstick or the precipitation of protein by addition of an acid to urine.[2] The familiar dipstick test is a convenient colorimetric assay which relies on the ability of proteins, particularly albumin, to alter the color of an acid-base indicator impregnated within a paper strip when the pH is maintained at a constant level. The color change is roughly proportional to the urinary protein concentration, varying from 0 (yellow) to 4+ (deep blue) with the following approximate estimations of protein concentration: trace = 10 mg/dl; 1+ = 30 mg/dl; 2+ = 100 mg/dl; 3+ = 300 mg/dl; and 4+ = 1000 mg/dl.

Protein precipitation techniques, including precipitation with either sulfosalicylic acid, heat and acetic acid, or concentrated nitric acid, rely on the somewhat subjective interpretation of turbidity induced when these agents react with urinary protein. Estimations of turbidity are also graded on a 0 (no precipitate) to 4+ (heavy flocculation) scale. Although less convenient than the dipstick test, the precipitation tests are more sensitive, detecting protein concentrations as low as 3 to 5 mg/dl. The precipitation tests are also more sensitive than the dipstick test in detecting nonalbumin proteins such as immunoglobulin light chains. Precipitation methods are probably best employed to corroborate a questionably positive dipstick test or to verify a false-positive dipstick reaction (see below). Commonly employed precipitation techniques and their interpretation are described in detail in the Appendix at the end of this chapter.

Semiquantitative tests for proteinuria are useful for screening, but their diagnostic utility is limited by relatively frequent false-positive and false-negative results. Furthermore, these tests do not provide an accurate assessment of the magnitude of protein excretion in patients with heavy proteinuria, so that they are generally unreliable in monitoring the effects of therapy.

False-Positive Semiquantitative Tests for Proteinuria

Table 1–2 lists some of the common causes of false-positive semiquantitative tests for urinary protein. Patients excreting small volumes of highly concentrated urine are among those most likely to demonstrate false-positive reactions. For example, a patient excreting 500 ml of urine per day with a daily protein excretion of 100 mg will have a urinary protein concentration of 20 mg/dl. Under these circumstances, semiquantitative tests would detect trace to 1+ protein, even though excretion of 100 mg of protein per day is quite normal. Thus, a false-positive result should be suspected when a trace to 1+ dipstick reading is observed in a highly concentrated urine specimen (specific gravity >1.025).

Patients with gross hematuria or pyuria may have false-positive tests for proteinuria resulting from the breakdown of the cellular elements into their proteinaceous components. In urologic conditions accompanied by hematuria and pyuria (e.g., urolithiasis, urinary tract neoplasms, or acute bacterial infections), proteinuria may result in part from the exudation of serum proteins at the pathologic site. Although the urine indeed contains protein under these conditions, the positive tests do not reliably indicate renal parenchymal injury.

When urine is highly alkaline (i.e., pH > 8), the dipstick test may yield a false-positive value because the buffer component of the indicator dye is overwhelmed by an actual shift in pH. Such highly alkaline urine specimens are encountered almost exclusively in patients with urinary tract infections due to urea-splitting organisms.[3] In such cases, a false-positive dipstick reading can be corroborated by a negative precipitation test since the precipitation methods are not affected by changes in urine pH.

Discrepancies between the dipstick and precipitation tests may also provide clues to false-positive tests in patients exposed to radiographic contrast materials or to high doses of certain antibiotics including cephalosporins, penicillins, and sulfonamide.[4-6] In these cases, precipitation tests for proteinuria may be false-positive, but the dipstick test remains negative (see Table 1–2).

TABLE 1–2.—SOME CAUSES OF FALSE-POSITIVE SEMIQUANTITATIVE TESTS FOR PROTEINURIA

CAUSE	DIPSTICK METHOD	PRECIPITATION METHODS
Highly concentrated urine	+	+
Gross hematuria or pyuria	+	+
Highly alkaline urine (pH > 8)	+	−
Radiographic contrast agents	−	+
High urinary levels of penicillins or cephalosporins	−	+
Sulfonamide metabolites in urine	−	+

False-Negative Semiquantitative Tests for Proteinuria

False-negative results are uncommon with the dipstick or precipitation tests for proteinuria and occur chiefly when these tests are performed on extremely dilute urine. For example, a patient excreting 4000 ml of urine per day with a daily protein excretion of 300 mg will have a urinary protein concentration of 7.5 mg/dl. The dipstick test may be negative even though excretion of 300 mg of protein per day is abnormally high.

The dipstick may also yield false-negative results due to the relative insensitivity of the indicator dye to nonalbumin proteins. The major clinical implication of this phenomenon is the inability of the dipstick to detect immunoglobulin light chains (i.e., Bence-Jones protein) in the urine of patients with multiple myeloma. Protein precipitation methods are more sensitive to immunoglobulins and other nonalbumin proteins. Bence-Jones protein can also be detected by gently heating a urine sample in a test tube. At 50 to 60°C, the protein forms a precipitate which dissolves on boiling and reappears as the urine cools. This simple test is unreliable in the presence of other urinary proteins. Urinary immunoelectrophoresis is usually required for definitive identification and quantitation of light chains. Detection of small quantities of Bence-Jones protein by immunoelectrophoresis may be possible only after the urine is concentrated 50- to 100-fold by repeated centrifugation.

Quantitative Assays for Urine Protein

A number of methods are available to quantify urinary protein excretion, all of which are based on the precipitation of protein. The standard reference methods for urinary protein determination, including the Kjeldahl analysis for nitrogen and the biuret test, have coefficients of variation less than 2%. Such precision is rarely warranted for routine clinical analyses and simpler techniques are ordinarily employed. Most commonly, sulfosalicylic acid is added to an aliquot of urine and the turbidity, measured with a photometer or nephelometer, is compared to standard solutions containing known concentrations of protein (see Appendix). The measured protein concentration is multiplied by the total volume of the urine sample and reported as milligrams per unit of time. The sulfosalicylic method is adequate for clinical analyses but has a coefficient of variation as large as 20%.[7]

Lack of precision in the quantitation of urinary protein may result from variations in the analytic technique but more frequently reflects inaccuracies in the timed collection of urine samples. Twenty-four-hour urine samples are most commonly employed for quantitative analyses. Providing the patient with a standard set of instructions helps to minimize collection errors. The patient should be instructed to discard the first morning void on the day of collection. All subsequent voided specimens, up to and including the first morning void on the following day, should be transferred immediately from a collection bottle to a common container.

The adequacy of a 24-hour urine collection can be ascertained by simultaneously measuring urinary creatinine excretion, based on the presumption that creatinine excretion is relatively constant and proportional to the patient's muscle mass, varying less than 15% on a day-to-day basis. The normal range for creatinine excretion in young men is 16 to 26 mg/kg of body weight/day, and in young women 12 to 24 mg/kg of body weight/day. Creatinine excretion declines steadily with age, accompanying a steady decline in muscle mass, so that patients beyond the age of 70 may excrete as little as 8 mg/kg of body weight/day. Because of these wide variations in normal creatinine excretion, determination of urinary creatinine provides only a rough guideline to the adequacy of a 24-hour urine collection when applied to a single specimen. On the other hand, measurement of urinary creatinine is quite helpful in assessing the adequacy of serial specimens obtained from the same patient over relatively short periods of time.

Recent studies suggest that determination of a urinary protein/creatinine ratio in single, voided urine samples correlates well with the quantity of protein measured in timed urine collections.[8, 9] In the presence of stable renal function, a urinary protein/creatinine ratio of more than 3.5 (mg/mg) correlates well with "nephrotic-range" proteinuria (i.e., greater than 3.5 grams of protein per day). A ratio of less than 0.2 suggests normal urinary protein excretion[8] (Fig 1–1). Although this convenient technique may be suitable for screening, its value in monitoring the effects of therapy in patients with heavy proteinuria remains to be proved.

The quantity of protein detected in normal urine varies with the analytical method employed but, on average, normal subjects excrete 50 to 100 mg of protein per 24 hours. One hundred fifty milligrams of protein per day is generally regarded as the upper limit of normal.

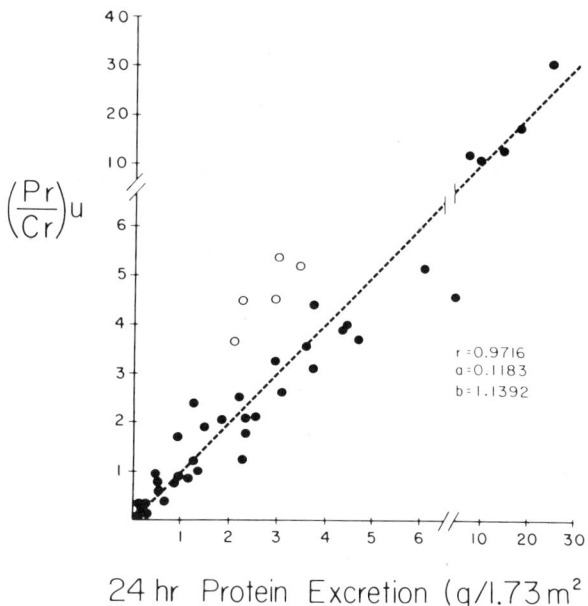

Fig 1–1.—Ratio of urinary protein to creatinine concentration [*(Pr)/(Cr)u*] of random, single, voided urine samples expressed as a function of 24-hour urinary protein excretion. The *five open circles* denote values for patients who had a protein/creatinine ratio of more than 3.5 and a protein excretion rate of less than 3.5 gm per 24 hours per 1.73 m^2. (Reprinted from Ginsberg et al., by permission of the *New England Journal of Medicine* 309:1543, 1983.)

APPROACH TO THE "HEALTHY" PATIENT WITH A POSITIVE TEST FOR URINE PROTEIN

Population surveys using semiquantitative methods to screen for proteinuria in apparently healthy subjects have found a prevalence of proteinuria ranging from 1% to 26%.[10] False-positive tests undoubtedly account for a substantial portion of these cases. A number of studies in military recruits and college students suggest that a positive test for proteinuria is most often an isolated and transient finding, with disappearance of proteinuria within days after the initial positive test. The term *benign transient proteinuria* has been adopted to describe this phenomenon. Patients with benign transient proteinuria virtually never have serious underlying renal disease and their long-term prognosis is excellent.

Given these considerations, when an apparently healthy patient has a 1+ or greater semiquantitative test for protein, the test should be repeated on one or two additional random urine samples before pursuing a more extensive investigation. If the semiquantitative tests are persistently positive, definitive evaluation requires the collection of a 24-hour urine specimen to verify and quantify the proteinuria. In addition, a persistently positive test for urine protein warrants a few preliminary laboratory tests to exclude overt renal disease. As a minimum, initial tests should include measurement of the blood urea nitrogen (BUN), a serum creatinine concentration, or creatinine clearance to estimate glomerular filtration rate, the best overall index of renal function. In addition, a complete urinalysis should be performed, including microscopic examination of the sediment from a freshly voided specimen. The presence of casts containing formed cellular elements is a reliable indicator of parenchymal renal disease. The discovery of red blood cell casts, in particular, virtually assures the presence of an underlying glomerular disease. Examination of the urine sediment should also include a search for free lipid droplets or oval fat bodies which exhibit characteristic negative birefringence when viewed with a polarizing lens. As discussed in Chapter 3, lipiduria occurs commonly in heavy proteinuric states. The discovery of lipids in the urinalysis of a patient with a positive test for urinary protein provides an early clue to the presence of heavy proteinuria and increases the likelihood of an underlying glomerulopathy. Regardless of whether overt renal disease is suspected on the basis of preliminary tests, further evaluation and management of the patient with a persistently positive semiquantitative test for urinary protein requires quantitation of protein excretion in a timed urine collection.

CLASSIFICATION OF PROTEINURIC STATES

Recognition of both quantitative and qualitative patterns of protein excretion is critical in assessing the presence and severity of renal disease and in managing the proteinuric patient. A simple classification scheme for various patterns of urinary protein excretion is shown in Table 1–3.

Intermittent Proteinuria

Intermittent proteinuria consists of an increase in protein excretion above normal in some, but not all urine specimens on repeated testing. In this category we include patients with *benign transient pro-*

teinuria which has been defined above. Also included in this category are patients with *functional proteinuria* which is defined as excessive excretion of urinary protein in the absence of parenchymal renal disease. Table 1–4 lists some of the more common causes of functional proteinuria. The pathophysiology of functional proteinuria remains incompletely understood, but renal vasoconstriction appears to be a common denominator among the disparate conditions listed in Table 1–4. As discussed in Chapter 2, a reduction in renal blood flow appears to facilitate the diffusion of albumin and other macromolecules across an intact glomerular capillary wall. Proteinuria can be produced in many normal subjects who adopt a posture of extreme lordosis. This phenomenon is most readily demonstrated in young patients,[11] and may reflect passive renal venous congestion resulting from compression of the inferior vena cava against the spine. A unique form of functional proteinuria occurs in patients receiving intravenous infusions of albumin or other plasma proteins. Because the glomerular capillary wall is relatively but not absolutely impermeable to circulating macromolecules, infusions of plasma proteins may result in excessive urinary protein excretion by increasing the concentration gradient for these proteins across the glomerular capillary membrane.

Functional proteinuria has been detected in as many as 10% of patients admitted to a general medical service.[12] The key to the management of the patient with functional proteinuria lies in the recognition of the underlying pathologic or physiologic disturbance. In the absence of underlying renal disease, urinary protein excretion typically returns to normal after recovery from the precipitating disorder. Among the conditions listed in Table 1–4, exercise, fever, and exposure to severe cold rarely increase urinary protein excretion more than threefold,[13, 14] so that quantitative analysis usually reveals less than 500 mg of protein per day. Greater amounts of urinary protein are occasionally detected in patients with severe congestive heart failure,[15] but heart failure alone rarely accounts for more than 1 to

TABLE 1–3.—CLASSIFICATION OF PROTEINURIC STATES

Intermittent
  Benign transient proteinuria
  Functional proteinuria
  Postural (orthostatic) proteinuria
Persistent
  Asymptomatic proteinuria
  Heavy proteinuria with or without the nephrotic syndrome

TABLE 1–4.—COMMON CAUSES OF FUNCTIONAL PROTEINURIA

High fever
Strenuous exercise
Exposure to cold
Infusions of norepinephrine
Congestive heart failure
Severe lordotic posture
Infusions of albumin or plasma protein ("overflow" proteinuria)

2 grams of urinary protein per day. Because all of the conditions listed in Table 1–4 may exacerbate proteinuria in patients with underlying renal disease, protein excretion exceeding 2 grams per day in these settings should always raise the concern of underlying renal parenchymal disease. With lesser amounts of proteinuria, an investigation for underlying renal disease should be pursued only if proteinuria persists after resolution of the precipitating disorder.

In most patients with proteinuria, protein excretion is typically greater in the upright than in the recumbent position. This phenomenon, which may be related to renal hemodynamic alterations accompanying changes in posture, should be differentiated from true *postural proteinuria* (or *orthostatic proteinuria*), a specific pattern of proteinuria in which excessive protein excretion occurs only in the upright posture. Patients with postural proteinuria have a normal excretion of protein when they are recumbent. As many as 20% of young adults with a positive test for urine protein on routine urinalysis demonstrate this pattern.[16] Daily protein excretion in patients with postural proteinuria is usually less than 1 gram.

The pathophysiology of postural proteinuria is also poorly understood. This pattern is often detected during the resolving stages of acute glomerulonephritis, but occurs more commonly in patients with no other clinical evidence of overt renal disease. In the latter group of patients, renal biopsy studies have generally demonstrated either normal histologic findings or mild mesangial proliferation. The major clinical significance of detecting this pattern of proteinuria lies in the excellent prognosis associated with reproducible postural proteinuria. Most long-term follow-up studies of patients with this disorder suggest that postural proteinuria remits slowly with time. More than 85% of patients exhibit complete remission from proteinuria after 20 years. Most importantly, renal insufficiency and hypertension occur rarely after 20 years of follow-up, even among those patients in whom postural proteinuria persists.[17]

To screen for postural proteinuria, the patient is instructed to void before retiring and to collect a morning urine specimen immediately upon arising. The dipstick test is performed on the morning sample and results are compared to those obtained on a random urine sample collected after several hours of upright posture. Definitive determination of postural proteinuria requires quantitative analyses in timed urine collections obtained in the upright and supine positions. The patient is instructed to begin a collection of urine while in the upright position after discarding the first morning void. Upon retiring, the patient records the number of hours spent in the upright position, voids before retiring to complete the upright collection, and then begins an overnight recumbent urine collection, usually consisting of a single voided specimen the following morning. Again, the number of hours spent in the recumbent position is recorded. The amount of protein measured in each sample is extrapolated to 24 hours. Patients have true postural proteinuria only if the extrapolated recumbent value falls within the normal range. For example:

A patient awakens at 8 A.M. and begins an upright urine collection. He retires at 12 midnight and sleeps in a recumbent position, rising to void a single overnight urine specimen at 8 A.M. the following morning.

The upright 16-hour urine specimen contains 300 mg of protein (=450 mg extrapolated to 24 hours). The recumbent 8-hour urine specimen contains 40 mg of protein (=120 mg extrapolated to 24 hours). Postural proteinuria is confirmed.

The management of patients with postural proteinuria is discussed in Chapter 6.

Persistent Proteinuria

Patients with persistent proteinuria exhibit excessive protein excretion in all urine samples on repeated testing, regardless of posture. Further categorization of patients with this pattern of proteinuria is based on quantitation of daily protein excretion. Patients with *asymptomatic proteinuria* usually excrete less than 3 grams of protein per day. They are asymptomatic in the sense that protein excretion of this magnitude is rarely associated with hypoalbuminemia or other clinical manifestations of the nephrotic syndrome. By contrast, patients with *heavy proteinuria* excrete more than 3 grams of protein per day and commonly exhibit some or all manifestations of the nephrotic syndrome including hypoalbuminemia, edema, hyperlipidemia and lipiduria. Important diagnostic and prognostic implications derive from this quantitative distinction. The detection of heavy proteinuria virtually assures the presence of an underlying glomerular disease, and prognosis depends critically on the specific glomerular histopathology. By contrast, patients with asymptomatic proteinuria may have an underlying glomerulopathy, but not infrequently have either a nonglomerular renal disease or normal histologic findings (see below). Not surprisingly, the prognosis of patients with asymptomatic proteinuria is extremely variable. There is no strong correlation between underlying histopathology and long-term renal prognosis in this group of proteinuric patients.

Patients with persistent asymptomatic proteinuria develop hypertension and renal failure more often than individuals without proteinuria. As many as 50% of patients with asymptomatic proteinuria develop hypertension within five years of follow-up[18] and as many as 20% develop renal insufficiency after 10 years.[16] The prognosis may be worse among patients in whom proteinuria is associated with microscopic hematuria.[19] Moreover, the association of hematuria with asymptomatic proteinuria increases the likelihood of an underlying renal parenchymal disease.[20]

Renal biopsy studies have revealed either normal histologic findings or mild mesangial proliferation in approximately 70% of patients with persistent asymptomatic proteinuria. Five to ten percent of such patients have one of a variety of tubulointerstitial diseases. The remaining 20% of patients have distinct glomerular lesions including membranous glomerulopathy, focal glomerulosclerosis, and membranoproliferative glomerulonephritis.[16] Renal biopsy can be performed to determine the precise histopathology in patients with asymptomatic proteinuria. Identification of specific histologic lesions may be helpful in assessing prognosis but provides little information of therapeutic value. For example, the discovery of focal glomerulosclerosis or membranoproliferative glomerulonephritis implies an unfavorable prognosis, but there are no established treatments for these diseases and their identification rarely influences patient management. With the exception of a single uncontrolled study suggesting a beneficial effect of corticosteroid therapy in patients with asymptomatic proteinuria and underlying membranous glomerulopathy,[21] few prospective studies have examined the effects of specific drug therapy (i.e., steroids or cytotoxic drugs) on the outcome of patients with asymptomatic proteinuria and glomerular disease. Until such studies are performed, renal biopsy is not justified as a routine procedure in patients with persistent asymptomatic proteinuria. Management of these patients is discussed further in Chapter 6.

Patients with heavy proteinuria and the nephrotic syndrome are broadly categorized as having either primary ("idiopathic") or secondary forms of the disorder. Because the clinical features of nephrotic syndrome often are the same whether the disorder is caused by primary renal disease or secondary to systemic illness, the physician is obliged to consider the secondary forms of nephrotic syndrome in all patients presenting with heavy proteinuria. The histopathology, clinical characteristics, prognosis, and management of patients with the nephrotic syndrome are discussed in detail in Chapters 3 through 5.

APPENDIX

Semiquantitative Precipitation Tests for Detection of Proteinuria

Interpretation of turbidity induced by the sulfosalicylic acid, or heat and acetic acid methods is based on the following scale:

GRADE	APPROXIMATE PROTEIN CONCENTRATION	TURBIDITY
0	<5 mg/dl	None
Trace	5 mg/dl	Faint turbidity viewed against a black background
1+	10 to 30 mg/dl	Small amount
2+	40 to 200 mg/dl	Moderate amount
3+	200 to 500 mg/dl	Heavy amount
4+	>500 mg/dl	Heavy flocculation

Sulfosalicylic Acid Method

1. Place 5 ml of urine in a test tube.
2. Add 3 drops of 20% sulfosalicylic acid.
3. Mix and estimate turbidity.

Heat and Acetic Acid Method

1. If urine is cloudy, centrifuge or filter first.
2. Place 5 ml of clear urine in a test tube.
3. Boil urine over a flame.

4. Add 3 drops of glacial acetic acid.
5. Re-boil and estimate turbidity.

Quantitative Sulfosalicylic Acid Turbidity Test

1. Pipette 2.5 ml of urine into a test tube.
2. Add 7.5 ml of 3% sulfosalicylic acid.
3. Mix, then let stand for ten minutes.
4. Compare the turbidity with known standards prepared from solutions containing 10, 20, 30, 40, 50, 75, and 100 mg of albumin/dl and estimate the concentration of the unknown specimen. If the unknown specimen contains more than 100 mg of protein/dl, dilute the urine and repeat the test.

REFERENCES

1. McKenzie J.K., Patel R., McQueen E.G.: The excretion rate Tamm-Horsfall urinary mucoprotein in normals and in patients with renal disease. *Aust. N. Z. J. Med.* 13:32, 1964.
2. Kassirer J.P., Gennari F.J.: Laboratory evaluation of renal function, in Earley L.E., Gottschalk C.W. (eds.): *Strauss and Welt's Diseases of the Kidney*. Boston, Little, Brown & Co., 1979, pp. 64–65.
3. Huntsman R.H., Liddell J.: The erroneous diagnosis of proteinuria due to bacterial contamination. *Guys Hospital Reports* 109:179, 1960.
4. Levy M., Elliakim M.: Urinary precipitate during cephalothin-cephaloridine treatment. *J.A.M.A.* 219:908, 1972.
5. Andreoli S.P., Kleiman M.B., Glick M.R., et al.: Nafcillin, pseudo-proteinuria, and hypokalemic alkalosis. *J. Pediatr.* 97:841, 1980.
6. Jensen H., Henriksen K.: Proteinuria in non-renal infectious disease. *Acta Med. Scand.* 196:75, 1974.
7. Henry R.J., Sobel C., Segalove M.: Turbidometric determination of proteins with sulfosalicylic and trichloroacetic acids. *Proc. Soc. Exp. Biol. Med.* 92:748, 1956.
8. Ginsberg J.M., Chang B.S., Materese R.A., Garella S.: Use of single voided urine samples to estimate quantitative proteinuria. *N. Engl. J. Med.* 309:1543, 1983.
9. Shaw A.B., Risdon P., Lewis-Jackson J.D.: Protein creatinine index and Albustix in assessment of proteinuria. *Br. Med. J.* 287:929, 1983.
10. Wolman I.J.: The incidence, causes and intermittency of proteinuria in young men. *Am. J. Med. Sci.* 210:86, 1945.
11. Bull G.M.: Postural proteinuria. *Clin. Sci.* 7:77, 1948.
12. Reuben D.B., Wachtel T.J., Brown P., et al.: Transient proteinuria in emergent medical admissions. *N. Engl. J. Med.* 306:1031, 1982.
13. Castenford J., Mossfeldt F., Piscator M.: Effect of prolonged heavy exercise on kidney function and urinary protein excretion. *Acta Physiol. Scand.* 70:194, 1967.
14. Hemmingsen L., Skaarup P.: Urinary excretion of ten plasma proteins in patients with febrile diseases. *Acta Med. Scand.* 201:359, 1977.
15. Albright R., Brensilver J., Cortell S.: Proteinuria in congestive heart failure. *Am. J. Nephrol.* 3:272, 1983.
16. Abuelo J.G.: Proteinuria: diagnostic principles and practices. *Ann. Intern. Med.* 98:186, 1983.
17. Springberg P.D., Garrett L.E., Thompson A.L., et al.: Fixed and reproducible or-

thostatic proteinuria: results of a 20-year follow up study. *Ann. Intern. Med.* 97:516, 1982.
18. King S.E.: Diastolic hypertension and chronic proteinuria. *Am. J. Cardiol.* 9:669, 1962.
19. Antoine B., Symvoulidis A., Dardenna M.: La stabilite evolutive des etats de proteinuric permanente isolee. *Nephron* 6:526, 1969.
20. Chen B.T.M., Ooi B., Tan K., et al.: Comparative studies of asymptomatic proteinuria and hematuria. *Arch. Intern. Med.* 134:901, 1974.
21. Kobayashi Y., Tateno S., Shigematsu H., et al.: Prednisone treatment in non-nephrotic patients with idiopathic membranous nephropathy. *Nephron* 30:210, 1982.

2 Mechanisms of Proteinuria

UNDERSTANDING THE MECHANISMS underlying excessive urinary protein excretion provides a basis for the diagnosis and management of proteinuric patients. In this chapter we first review those features of normal renal structure and function that account for the excretion of negligible amounts of urinary protein in health. We then consider pathogenetic mechanisms of excessive urinary protein excretion in glomerular and nonglomerular renal diseases. Because immunologically mediated glomerular diseases constitute an important subset of renal diseases associated with heavy proteinuria, we include a brief review of immunologic mechanisms of glomerular injury. Finally, we consider possible mechanisms underlying functional forms of proteinuria.

PROTEIN-HANDLING BY THE NORMAL KIDNEY

The formation of urine begins at the glomerular capillary membrane with the separation of approximately 20% of plasma entering the capillary lumen into a nearly ideal ultrafiltrate that enters the proximal nephron. Despite its very low resistance to the flow of water and low molecular weight substances, the glomerular capillary membrane greatly impedes the filtration of all but the smallest of circulating macromolecules. Evidence from micropuncture studies in animals suggests that the normal glomerular capillary wall is relatively, but not absolutely, impermeable to circulating proteins. In rats, direct collections of the glomerular filtrate by micropuncture have revealed concentrations of albumin as low as 0.1 mg/dl in the early proximal tubule.[1] Since the albumin concentration in the capillary lumen is at least 3000 mg/dl, the concentration gradient for albumin across the rat glomerular capillary membrane may be as high as 30,000:1.

The amount of protein that crosses the human glomerular capillary remains a matter of speculation. If data from animal studies can be extrapolated to man, as little as 180 mg of albumin may leak across the glomerular capillary each day (presuming a normal glomerular filtration rate of 180 liters/day and a minimal albumin concentration of 0.1 mg/dl in the early proximal tubule). A more conservative estimate is that 500 to 2000 mg of albumin leaks across the normal human glomerulus each day. Considering the huge quantity of albumin in plasma coursing through the glomerular capillaries on a daily basis, it is clear that the relative impermeability of the glomerular capillary membrane to circulating macromolecules plays a major role in limiting the quantity of protein excreted in normal urine.

As is true of all substances excreted by the kidney, the quantity of protein in the final urine reflects a balance between the amount filtered through the glomerulus and the amounts secreted and reabsorbed by the renal tubule (Fig 2–1). It is theoretically possible that plasma proteins are transported from peritubular capillaries across

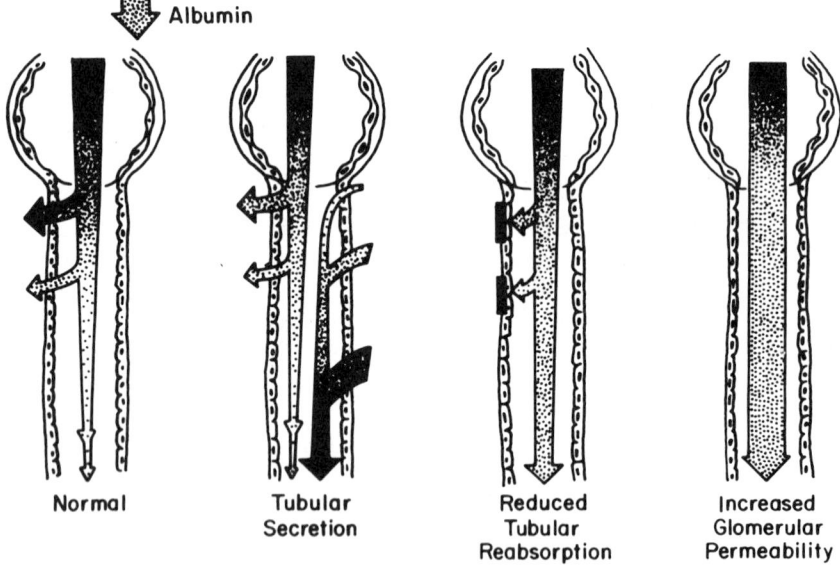

Fig 2–1.—Theoretical mechanisms of urinary protein excretion. Under normal conditions, small amounts of protein leak across the glomerular capillary membrane and are partially reabsorbed by renal tubular cells. In theory, urinary protein excretion could be increased by tubular secretion of protein, reduced tubular reabsorption of filtered protein, or by increased permeability of the capillary membrane. (See text for details.)

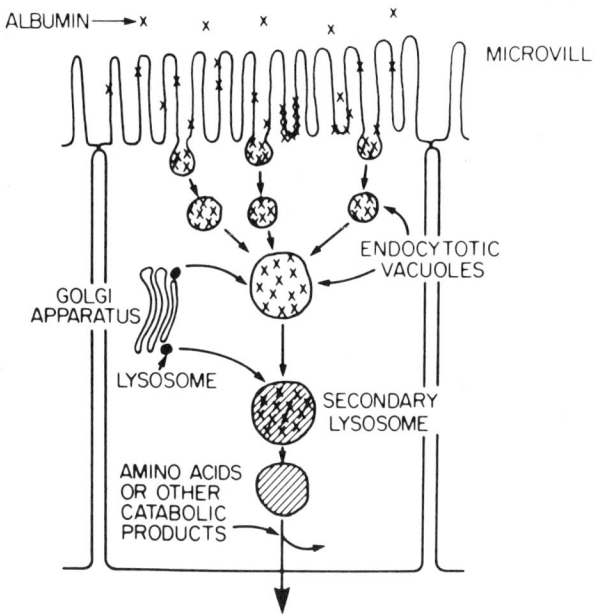

Fig 2–2.—Tubular reabsorption and catabolism of albumin. Filtered albumin molecules *(X)* attach to the brush border of proximal tubular cells. Protein molecules are absorbed by endocytosis; small endocytotic vacuoles fuse to form larger ones. Lysosomes then fuse with the vacuoles and protein is digested into constituent amino acids that return to the circulation. (From Earley L.E., Forland M.: Nephrotic syndrome, in Earley L.E., Gottshalk C.W. (eds.): *Strauss and Welt's Diseases of the Kidney.* Boston, Little, Brown & Co., 1979, p. 776. Used by permission.)

tubular epithelium into the tubular lumen, but there is little evidence for tubular secretion of albumin or other circulating macromolecules. Tubular reabsorption of proteins that leak across the glomerular capillary membrane has been clearly demonstrated, however. Reabsorption of filtered albumin occurs through a process of endocytosis that occurs at the luminal surface of the proximal tubule. Studies employing radiolabeled albumin suggest that little, if any, of the reabsorbed protein is returned intact to the circulation.[2] Following intratubular injection, labeled albumin binds to the brush border membrane of the proximal tubular cells. Vacuoles subsequently form along the luminal surface of the cells, engulfing the isotope. As these vacuoles migrate into the cell, entrapped protein molecules are subject to hydrolytic cleavage by lysosomal enzymes (Fig 2–2). Methods are not available to precisely quantitate the magnitude of this reabsorptive process; however, the presence of small quantities of plasma proteins in the urine of normal subjects suggests that the process is never complete.

A similar process of glomerular filtration and tubular reabsorption characterizes the normal renal handling of smaller proteins and peptides. Included among this class of compounds are immunoglobulin light chains, various microglobulins, and a number of peptide hormones including insulin, glucagon, and parathyroid hormone. Largely because of their smaller size (see below), these compounds filter across the glomerular capillary wall more readily than albumin or high molecular weight globulins. Small linear peptides are hydrolyzed directly by brush border enzymes at the luminal membrane, followed by reabsorption of constituent amino acids.[3] Larger peptides are absorbed by vacuolization and intracellular degradation. In contrast to the minor role that the normal kidney plays in the catabolism of albumin, smaller molecular weight proteins are extensively reabsorbed and degraded by the renal tubule. Not surprisingly, renal tubular dysfunction or disease may alter the catabolism of these substances and enhance their excretion in the urine as intact molecules.

A number of factors modify the amount of protein normally excreted in the urine. Presuming that the concentration gradient for albumin across the glomerular capillary membrane is constant, the amount of albumin delivered to the early proximal tubule can be altered simply by changing the plasma albumin concentration. Thus, "overflow" proteinuria occurs when the plasma albumin concentration is raised sufficiently by intravenous infusion of albumin. Variations in renal hemodynamics also modify normal urinary protein excretion. When renal plasma flow is reduced but the glomerular filtration rate remains normal, the resulting increase in the fraction of plasma filtered increases the concentration of plasma proteins toward the efferent end of the glomerular capillary and favors the movement of weakly permeant proteins across the glomerular capillary wall into the proximal nephron. A number of studies also suggest that increments in the glomerular filtration rate of single nephrons may directly alter glomerular permselectivity by increasing the transglomerular flux of circulating macromolecules.[4,5] Although this concept of glomerular "hyperfiltration" has been invoked most commonly as a pathogenetic factor accounting for proteinuria in chronic progressive renal disease, it is plausible that minor diurnal variations of glomerular filtration rate in the healthy kidney may slightly modify normal urinary protein excretion.

In summary, information about protein-handling by the normal kidney has been extrapolated largely from animal studies. The bulk of experimental evidence favors the concept that the glomerular capillary membrane is highly impermeable to most circulating plasma proteins. Small quantities of protein regularly leak across this membrane, the exact amount being modified to a minor degree by renal hemodynamic factors. Filtered proteins are partially reabsorbed by the proximal tubule, but small amounts of protein escape this process and are normally excreted in urine. Because the relative impermeability of the glomerulus appears to be the major factor limiting urinary protein excretion, the remainder of this section will focus on those properties of the normal glomerulus that account for restricted filtration of circulating macromolecules.

Size-Selective Properties of the Glomerulus

Clearance studies using various-sized macromolecules suggest that the normal glomerular capillary membrane behaves as a sieve that restricts filtration of solute molecules on the basis of their molecular weight and size. Dextran is a substance ideally suited for such clearance studies since its molecular weight and size can be varied intentionally over a wide range, and because it is neither secreted nor reabsorbed by renal tubular cells. Dextran clearance is conventionally expressed as a fraction of the clearance of inulin, a low molecular weight substance that is freely filtered across the glomerular capillary membrane. Using dextrans of increasing molecular size, it has been shown that fractional clearance progressively declines as the effective molecular radius of infused dextran molecules exceeds 20 Å, with virtually no excretion of dextran molecules having radii greater than 42 Å.[6] As early as 1953, investigators employing similar clearance techniques postulated that the walls of glomerular capillaries contained pores with an effective radius of approximately 45 Å.[7]

Ultrastructural characterization of the glomerular capillary membrane using electron microscopy reveals that the glomerular capillary wall is a complex, multilayered membrane that differs from capillary membranes in other vascular beds in a number of respects: (1) the endothelial fenestrae, measuring 500 to 1000 Å in width, are much larger than those of other fenestrated capillaries; (2) the basement membrane is considerably wider; (3) the outer adventitial layer of other capillaries is replaced by an elaborate epithelial layer consisting of interdigitating foot processes bridged by epithelial slit diaphragms (Fig 2–3). This characterization of glomerular ultrastructure fails to delineate the hypothetical pores predicted by clearance studies since both the endothelial fenestrae and the gaps between foot processes (averaging 250 Å in width) are too large to account for the restriction of macromolecules such as albumin which has an effective molecular radius of 36 Å.

Further attempts to establish a structural basis for glomerular permselectivity have employed electron microscopy following infusion of various electron-dense tracer molecules. Substances utilized for this purpose include either inherently electron-dense particulate tracers (e.g., ferritin or colloidal gold) or proteins (e.g., catalase, myeloperoxidase, lactoperoxidase) that can be visualized after a secondary enzymatic reaction yields electron-dense products. Early studies of this kind were performed with the assumption that the glomerular capillary wall is a size-selective porous filter and with the expectation that a sharp drop in the microscopically detected concentration of the tracer should occur at the level of the structure that restricts passage of the tracer. Numerous studies using a variety of tracers have failed to localize any single permeability barrier within the glomerular capillary wall. Instead, the ultrastructural site of tracer localization is quite variable, depending in part on the molecular weight and size of the molecule (Fig 2–4). For example, native horse-spleen ferritin (mo-

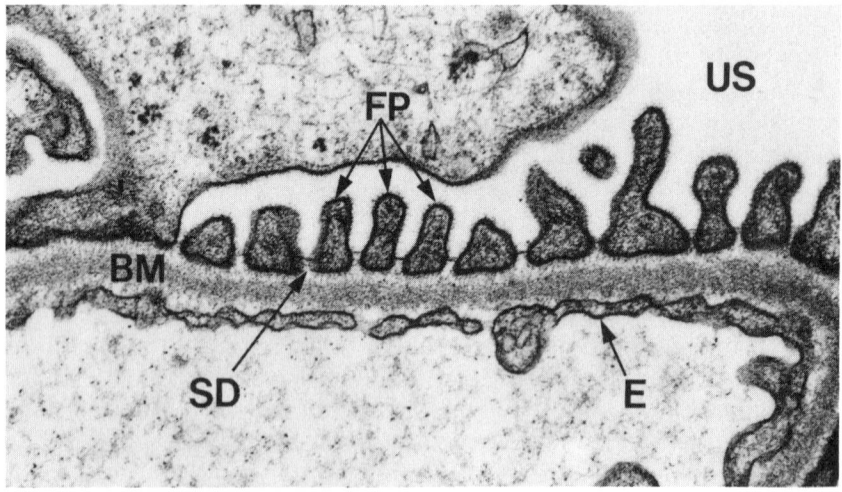

Fig 2–3.—Ultrastructure of the glomerular capillary membrane. *US* = urinary space; *BM* = basement membrane; *SD* = slit diaphragm; *FP* = epithelial foot processes; *E* = endothelium; ×39,000.

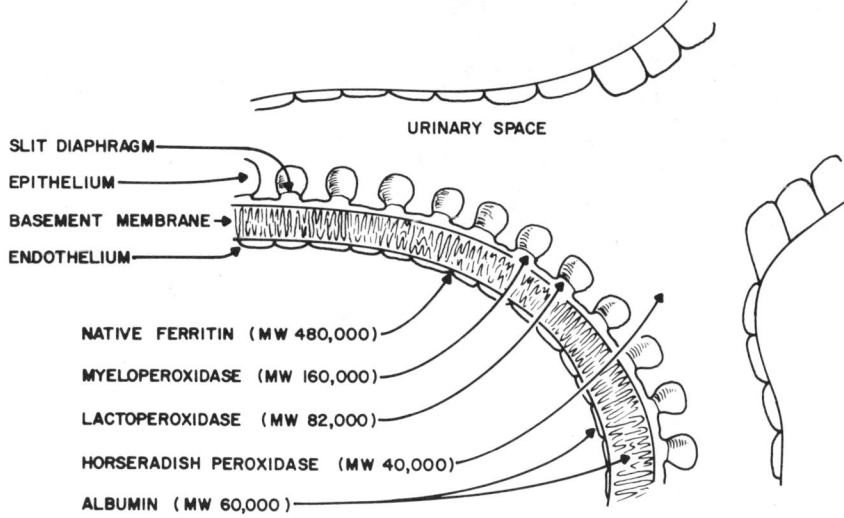

Fig 2–4.—Localization of various tracer proteins in the glomerular capillary membrane of normal kidneys.

lecular weight 480,000, effective radius 61 Å) is retarded at the level of the glomerular basement membrane.[8] Myeloperoxidase (molecular weight 160,000, effective radius 38 Å) and lactoperoxidase (molecular weight 82,000, effective radius 38 Å) penetrate the basement membrane and are hindered in the region of the epithelial slit diaphragm.[9, 10] Horseradish peroxidase (molecular weight 40,000, effective radius 30 Å) penetrates the entire capillary wall and appears in the glomerular filtrate.[9, 11] These early observations failed to ascribe a major restrictive influence to any single component of the glomerular wall, but they did suggest that the glomerular capillary membrane is a coarse filter capable of size discrimination: the larger the macromolecule, the more proximal the site of restriction within the capillary wall.

More recent studies using endogenous serum albumin as a tracer probe raise questions about the validity of the hypothesis that the glomerular capillary is a simple size-selective filter. Albumin (molecular weight 60,000, effective radius 36 Å) is smaller than myeloperoxidase or lactoperoxidase, but its filtration is retarded more proximally at the level of the capillary endothelium and proximal basement membrane[12] (see Fig 2–4). This observation suggests that the glomerular capillary membrane does not restrict filtration of circulating macromolecules solely on the basis of size.

Charge-Selective Properties of the Glomerulus

Several lines of evidence indicate that molecular charge is an additional determinant of the filtration of macromolecules across the glomerular capillary. The histochemical affinity of the normal glomerular capillary membrane for cationic reagents such as alcian blue and colloidal iron suggests that the glomerulus is rich in anionic sites that impart a net negative charge to the capillary wall. The effect of this negatively charged electrostatic barrier on glomerular permselectivity has been demonstrated in studies which show a reduced renal clearance of negatively charged dextrans as compared to that of neutral dextrans of the same size.[13] Conversely, cationically charged dextrans are cleared more readily than neutral dextrans of comparable size.[14] The existence of a charge-selective barrier to macromolecular filtration is further supported by studies employing highly charged, electron-dense tracers. In such studies, cationically charged tracers penetrate the glomerular capillary wall more readily than neutral or anionic tracers of the same size.[15,16] Thus, the normal glomerular capillary membrane can be viewed as a negatively charged electrostatic barrier that retards the filtration of circulating polyanions while facilitating the filtration of circulating polycations. Given these considerations, it is understandable that the filtration of albumin is restricted to a much greater extent than would be predicted from considerations of size alone. At normal plasma pH, albumin has a net negative charge and therefore permeates the capillary wall's electrostatic barrier less readily than neutral or cationic molecules of comparable size.

The biochemical nature of the anionic sites within the glomerulus has been a subject of active investigation. Two major classes of anionic substances account for the negative charge of the glomerular capillary wall. The glomerular endothelium, basement membrane, and epithelial foot processes contain *glycoproteins* with numerous sialic acid and acidic amino acid residues. In addition, the basement membrane is abundantly endowed with various *proteoglycans* rich in anionic sulfate groups. Proteoglycans consist of glycosaminoglycan chains linked to protein molecules. Although the glomerular basement membrane contains a number of glycosaminoglycans bound to a backbone of Type IV collagen, biochemical analyses indicate that heparan sulfate is the principal glycosaminoglycan in the basement membrane.[17,18] Glycoprotein moeities may play an important role in maintaining the structural integrity of epithelial foot processes and other components of the glomerular capillary wall; however, recent studies suggest that proteoglycans within the basement membrane are more crucial to the electrostatic barrier function of the glomerulus.[19-21] Indeed, enzymatic digestion of heparan sulfate with heparinase increases the permeability of albumin across the capillary wall.[21] It remains unclear whether loss of heparan sulfate under these circumstances causes proteinuria by exerting a direct effect on charge or by altering the structural integrity, and thus the size-selectivity, of the basement membrane.

The discovery of charge-selective properties of the glomerular capillary wall makes it unreasonable to ascribe a major filtration barrier function to any single structural component of the glomerulus and may account for the inability of investigators to identify the precise anatomical counterpart of the functional "pores" suggested by early clearance studies. It seems likely that some combined effect of the charge-selective barrier with the size-selective properties of the glomerular capillary membrane accounts for the generation by the normal kidney of a glomerular ultrafiltrate that is nearly free of plasma proteins.

MECHANISMS OF PROTEINURIA IN RENAL DISEASE

The above consideration of protein-handling by the normal kidney provides a basis for understanding the pathophysiology of proteinuria in disease states. In theory, three mechanisms could account for excessive urinary protein excretion in renal disease: (1) enhanced tubular secretion of plasma proteins; (2) reduced tubular reabsorption of proteins that leak across the glomerular capillary; or (3) increased permeability of the glomerular capillary membrane to circulating macromolecules. There is no direct evidence to suggest that tubular secretion of protein plays a significant role in urinary protein excretion in health or disease. Reduced tubular reabsorption of filtered protein probably accounts for the enhanced excretion of peptides and small molecular weight proteins in patients with certain tubulointerstitial renal diseases (see below); however, even complete failure to reabsorb the small amount of albumin that normally escapes into the proximal tubule could not by itself account for the albumin excretion rates typical of patients with renal parenchymal disease. The preponderance of evidence indicates that increased permeability of the glomerular capillary membrane is the major disturbance responsible for proteinuria in renal disease.

Patterns of Protein Excretion in Renal Disease

Three general categories of proteinuria have been defined on the basis of electrophoretic analyses of urinary proteins in patients with renal disease: glomerular, tubular, and overproduction proteinuria (Fig 2–5). In *glomerular proteinuria,* the electrophoretic pattern of urinary proteins mirrors that of serum proteins so that albumin is the predominant protein lost in the urine. Glomerular proteinuria is the most common pattern observed in patients with renal disease. It can be subdivided into either a "selective" or a "nonselective" pattern based on a comparison of the clearance of albumin with the clearance of larger molecular weight proteins. A selective pattern of proteinuria indicates that urinary protein consists largely of albumin, whereas a nonselective pattern indicates a relatively large amount of a high mo-

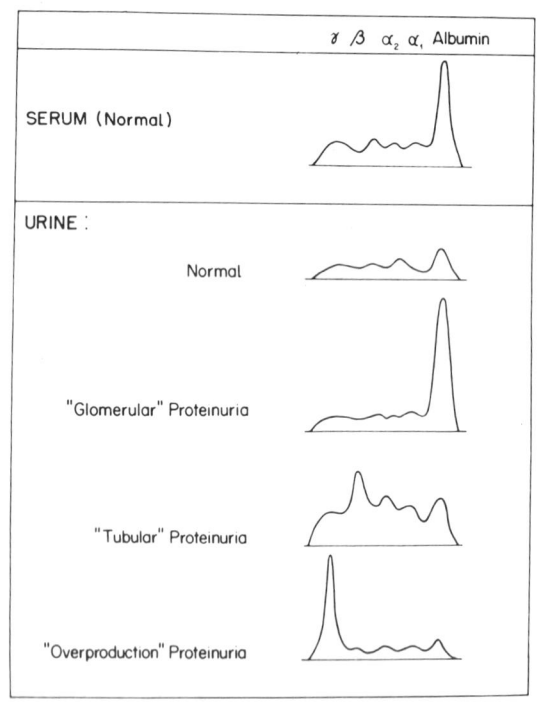

Fig 2–5.—Electrophoretic patterns of normal serum, normal urine, and of urines with three types of abnormal protein excretion. (From Kassirer J.P., Gennari F.J.: Laboratory evaluation of renal function, in Earley L.E., Gottshalk C.W. (eds.): *Strauss and Welt's Diseases of the Kidney.* Boston, Little, Brown & Co., 1979, p. 67. Used by permission.)

lecular weight, nonalbumin protein in the urine. In practice, selectivity is measured as the ratio of the renal clearance of IgG to the clearance of transferrin, a globulin with a molecular weight comparable to albumin. A clearance ratio for IgG/transferrin of less than 0.10 constitutes a "highly selective" pattern of glomerular proteinuria, while a clearance ratio greater than 0.30 defines a "poorly selective" pattern. As discussed below, the wide range of selectivity patterns among patients with proteinuria probably reflects differences in the molecular basis of proteinuria in various glomerulopathies. In certain clinical settings, determination of selectivity has important diagnostic and prognostic implications that affect management of the proteinuric patient (see Chapter 6).

Tubular proteinuria describes a pattern of abnormal protein excretion in which low molecular weight proteins such as light chains, lysozyme, and various microglobulins predominate over albumin. This pattern of proteinuria characterizes a diverse group of tubulointerstitial diseases including acute tubular necrosis, hereditary or acquired Fanconi syndrome, hypokalemic nephropathy, and Balkan nephropathy. A similar pattern may be found in patients with renal tubular damage secondary to infection, nephrotoxic agents, or transplant rejection. Tubular proteinuria results from impaired tubular reabsorption of low molecular weight proteins rather than from increased glomerular permeability. Indeed, the clearance rates for small proteins and peptides in patients with Fanconi syndrome approach the predicted filtration rates for these substances if the assumption is made that no tubular reabsorption occurs. The detection of increased quantities of low molecular weight urinary proteins such as lysozyme may aid in the diagnosis of various tubulointerstitial diseases.[22] Under most circumstances, however, tubular proteinuria accounts for only a negligible increase in daily urinary protein excretion. Furthermore, in chronic tubulointerstitial nephropathies, the pattern of proteinuria frequently shifts from a tubular to a glomerular pattern with progression of the disease. As will be discussed below, an increase in glomerular permeability to albumin and other circulating macromolecules is the major factor accounting for clinically significant proteinuria in both glomerular and nonglomerular renal diseases.

Overproduction proteinuria is characteristic of a group of nonrenal disorders in which proteinuria results from overproduction of low molecular weight plasma proteins that filter through the glomeruli, overload tubular reabsorptive capacity, and appear in the urine. This pattern of proteinuria is found most commonly in multiple myeloma patients who excrete immunoglobulin light chains. Another example of overproduction proteinuria is lysozymuria in patients with myelocytic leukemias.[23]

The Molecular Basis of Glomerular Proteinuria

At least two factors can theoretically account for the enhanced transglomerular passage of protein which accompanies glomerular injury: (1) an increase in the effective "pore" size or number of pores within the glomerular capillary membrane; and (2) changes in the electrostatic properties of the glomerular capillary wall. In addition, as discussed in the next section, disease-induced alterations in glomerular pressures and flows undoubtedly modify urinary protein excretion in both glomerular and nonglomerular renal diseases.

An alteration in the electrostatic barrier function of the glomerular capillary membrane appears to be the preeminent mechanism accounting for proteinuria in two widely studied experimental models of glomerulonephritis—nephrotoxic serum nephritis and puromycin-induced nephrosis. Albuminuria is a regular feature of both models. However, dextran clearance studies in these experimental models show that the fractional clearance of neutral dextran molecules equal in size to albumin is actually decreased from values in normal controls.[24, 25] The enhanced clearance of albumin and reduced clearance of comparably sized neutral dextrans in these experimental forms of glomerular disease cannot be explained by a change in effective pore size. Instead, data from such clearance studies strongly suggest that the underlying disease process somehow reduces the number of fixed glomerular anionic sites. Such a reduction in the net negative charge of the glomerular capillary wall would enhance the clearance of circulating polyanions while simultaneously retarding the clearance of neutral or cationic macromolecules. This hypothesis is supported by histochemical studies that demonstrate a great reduction in glomerular polyanion content in both of these experimental models.[26]

In human glomerular disease, proteinuria results from alterations in both the charge-selective and size-selective properties of the glomerulus, but the relative role played by each of these factors varies depending on the underlying glomerular histopathology. Histochemical studies demonstrate a reduction in glomerular polyanion content in a wide variety of human glomerulopathies,[27] suggesting that the attenuation of the net negative charge of the glomerular capillary may be a universal mechanism contributing to albuminuria in hu-

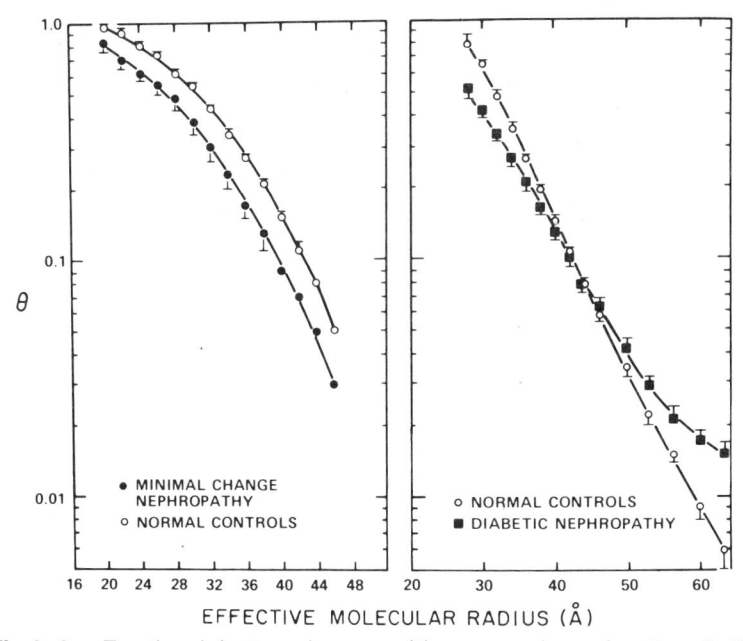

Fig 2–6.—Fractional dextran clearance (θ) expressed as a function of effective molecular radius in 10 patients with minimal change nephropathy *(closed circles, left panel)* and 16 patients with diabetic nephropathy *(closed squares, right panel)*, compared to that of normal controls *(open circles)*. In minimal change nephropathy, dextran clearance is impeded over a wide range of molecular radii. In diabetic nephropathy, clearance of small dextran molecules is impeded but clearance of large dextran molecules exceeds that of controls. (From Deen W.M., et al.: The glomerular barrier to macromolecules: theoretical and experimental considerations, in Brenner B.M., Stein J.H. (eds.): *Contemporary Issues in Nephrology.* New York, Churchill Livingstone, Inc., 1982, vol. 9, p. 22. Used by permission.)

man glomerular disease. The role of alterations in size-selectivity is more variable among the known glomerulopathies and appears to correlate with the extent of overt structural damage to the glomerular capillary membrane. At one end of the spectrum of human glomerular diseases is minimal change nephropathy, a disorder in which the glomerular architecture is well preserved (see Chapter 5). Dextran clearance studies in patients with this disorder yield results remarkably similar to those obtained in experimental nephrotoxic serum nephritis or puromycin-induced nephrosis (Fig 2–6). Data from such studies suggest that, in minimal change nephropathy, proteinuria results primarily from a disorder of electrostatic barrier function: the glomerulus retains its ability to discriminate molecular size but not molecular charge.[28] The clinical correlate of this isolated derangement in electrostatic barrier function is a highly selective pattern of proteinuria with a preponderance of albumin in the urine. At the other end of the spectrum is diabetic glomerulosclerosis, a disorder characterized by gross distortion of the glomerular capillary architecture (see Chapter 4). In patients with diabetic nephropathy, clearance of small neutral dextran molecules is lower than in normal subjects, reflecting a reduced negative charge of the glomerular capillary wall (see Fig 2–6). However, clearance of larger dextrans tends to be elevated above normal, suggesting that large pores develop within the glomerular capillary membrane in this disorder: the glomerulus loses its ability to discriminate both molecular size and molecular charge.[29] Albuminuria in diabetic nephropathy results in part from the loss of glomerular negative charge; larger nonalbumin proteins presumably leak through enlarged pores. Patients with diabetic nephropathy consequently exhibit a poorly selective pattern of glomerular proteinuria. For other glomerulopathies that fall within this spectrum of human glomerular diseases, it seems likely that proteinuria results from some combination of the effects of glomerular injury on both the size of pores and the charge on the capillary membrane.

Although alterations in charge and size-selectivity appear to be final common pathways accounting for glomerular proteinuria, the exact mechanisms leading to loss of negative charge or increments in pore size remain to be elucidated. It is tempting to speculate that humoral or cellular components of the immune system may directly alter the biochemical composition, and thus the charge, of the glomerular capillary wall in immunologically mediated glomerular diseases. For example, it has been postulated that the decrement in glomerular negative charge in minimal change nephropathy may be mediated by some humoral product of lymphocytes,[30, 31] but such a substance has yet to be identified. Much less is known about the mechanisms accounting for an increment in glomerular pore size. Recent studies suggest that the terminal components of the complement system may directly alter the structural integrity of the basement membrane in glomerular diseases mediated by immune-complex deposition and complement activation.[32] In those glomerulopathies characterized by overt structural damage to the glomerular capillary wall, frank disruptions of the basement membrane or glomerular epithelium may account for the large pores suggested by clearance studies.

MECHANISMS OF PROTEINURIA IN NONGLOMERULAR RENAL DISEASE: THE ROLE OF INTRARENAL HEMODYNAMIC FACTORS

The proteinuria observed in renal diseases that predominantly affect glomeruli is not unexpected. However, proteinuria also occurs in nonglomerular renal diseases. It is not unusual for protein excretion rates to range between 1 and 2 grams per day in patients with moderately advanced tubulointerstitial nephropathies. Decreased tubular reabsorption of filtered protein due to tubular dysfunction may contribute to excessive urinary protein excretion in such patients. However, albumin and high molecular weight globulins account for the bulk of urinary protein in advanced tubulointerstitial diseases, suggesting that alterations in glomerular function permit increased passage of plasma proteins across the glomerular capillary membrane—even in the absence of glomerular pathology.

Recent studies suggest that such functional alterations in glomerular permselectivity result from adaptive intrarenal hemodynamic changes that occur in residual nephrons when the total nephron population is reduced. One striking adaptive change that develops under these circumstances is a marked increase in the glomerular filtration rate of residual nephrons. This increase in single nephron glomerular filtration rate results from compensatory increases in glomerular plasma flow and transcapillary hydraulic pressure which serve to preserve whole kidney glomerular filtration rate and to maintain overall glomerulotubular balance. Increments in single nephron plasma flow and hydraulic pressure have been shown to increase the permeability of the glomerular capillary membrane to circulating proteins.[33, 34] Numerous experimental observations support the hypothesis that compensatory hyperfiltration in residual nephrons accounts for proteinuria in nonglomerular diseases. In normal rats, unilateral nephrectomy is followed by a 40% increase in the glomerular filtration rate of the remaining kidney and by an almost threefold increase in urinary protein excretion.[35] In animals with experimentally induced unilateral pyelonephritis, protein excretion increases fivefold when the nephron population is reduced by removing the normal contralateral kidney.[35]

The principles derived from these experimental observations probably apply to all chronic kidney diseases accompanied by a reduction in renal mass, regardless of whether the original disease process has primarily affected the glomeruli, blood vessels, tubules, or interstitium. In most patients with nonglomerular renal diseases and mild to moderate renal insufficiency, proteinuria results primarily from compensatory alterations in the hemodynamic determinants of glomerular filtration rate. In addition to the functional alterations in glomerular permselectivity which accompany chronic progressive renal disease, it has been postulated that compensatory residual nephron hyperfiltration may ultimately induce structural damage in residual glomeruli, leading to sclerosis of glomerular capillaries.[36] This hypothesis may account for the development of focal glomerulosclerosis and heavy proteinuria in some patients with advanced renal insufficiency due to tubulointerstitial diseases such as analgesic-abuse nephropathy and vesicoureteral reflux nephropathy.[37]

IMMUNOLOGIC MECHANISMS OF GLOMERULAR INJURY

Although excessive excretion of urinary protein is characteristic of most renal diseases, it should be obvious from the foregoing discussion that heavy proteinuria and the nephrotic syndrome occur almost exclusively in patients with renal diseases that primarily affect the glomeruli. The glomerulopathies have been categorized in several ways. First, by *clinical features,* i.e., according to the presenting clinical syndrome; second, by *morphology,* i.e., according to the integrated findings of light, immunofluorescence, and electron microscopy; third, by *etiology;* and finally, according to the *pathogenetic mechanisms.* Much of the remainder of this book will deal with the clinical features, histopathology, and etiology of various glomerulopathies associated with the nephrotic syndrome. In this section, we focus on pathogenetic mechanisms of glomerular injury. The pathogenesis of certain degenerative and hereditary glomerulopathies (e.g., diabetic glomerulosclerosis, congenital nephrotic syndrome, hereditary nephritis) remains to be elucidated. Since most of the glomerulopathies seen in clinical practice appear to be mediated by immunologic mechanisms, this section will concentrate on the mechanisms of glomerular capillary wall injury induced by immune-deposits.

Mechanisms of Glomerular Immune-Complex Formation

The majority of immunologically mediated glomerulopathies are associated with glomerular deposits of immunoglobulins and their accompanying antigens. Although antibody-antigen complexes may directly alter the structural integrity of the glomerular capillary wall, their proclivity to induce proteinuria more often results from the activation of secondary immune reactants such as complement, coagulation factors, and inflammatory cells. Immunologically mediated glomerular injury has traditionally been ascribed to one of two basic mechanisms of immune-deposit formation: (1) deposition of circulating antibodies to endogenous basement membrane antigens (antiglomerular basement membrane disease); or (2) deposition of circulating antibody-antigen complexes at various sites within the glomerulus (immune-complex glomerulonephritis). Antiglomerular basement membrane disease is manifested on immunofluorescence and electron microscopy by continuous or "linear" deposits of immunoglobulin along the basement membrane, whereas immune-complex glomerulonephritis produces "granular" deposits within the basement membrane or mesangium. This traditional categorization of immune glomerular injury has recently been expanded and modified. Furthermore, recent evidence suggests that cell-mediated immune mechanisms can also induce glomerular injury.

It is now clear that antibodies reacting with endogenous basement membrane antigens can produce both linear and granular immune-deposits, depending on the distribution of the antigen.[38] In most examples of human antiglomerular basement membrane disease, the circulating antibodies are heterogeneous, possessing reactivity to a number of antigenic determinants within the basement membrane. Thus, most cases of human antiglomerular basement membrane disease conform to the traditional theory, being manifest by linear deposition of immunoglobulins along the basement membranes. It remains unknown whether the generation of antiglomerular basement membrane antibodies represents a true autoimmune reaction or the normal immune response to exogenous antigens that cross-react with antigenic determinants in the basement membrane. Although animal models of antiglomerular basement membrane disease have provided a great deal of information regarding immunologically mediated proteinuria, this mechanism of immune-deposit formation accounts for less than 5% of human glomerular disease.

Glomerular trapping of circulating immune-complexes has long been accepted as the most common immunologic mechanism of renal injury, but the importance of this mechanism in the pathogenesis of glomerulonephritis has recently been questioned. Observations in experimental animals and in human diseases have provided evidence that immune-complexes containing nonglomerular antigens can produce a variety of morphologic forms of glomerular disease, including acute proliferative lesions as well as chronic diseases with prolifera-

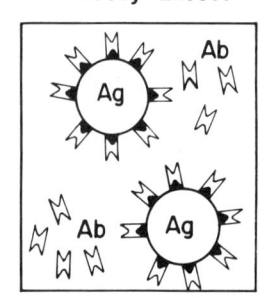

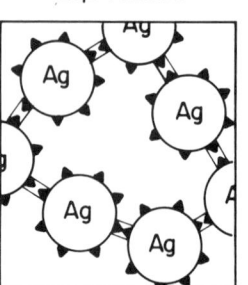

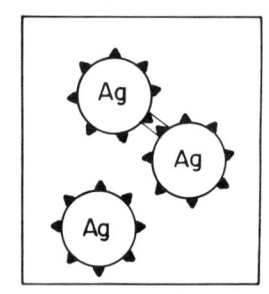

Fig 2–7.—Size of circulating immune-complexes as determined by relative proportions of antibody and antigen. Small, poorly precipitable complexes form with either antibody or antigen excess. Large precipitable complexes form with antibody-antigen equivalence. (Modified from McIntosh R.M., et al.: Immunologic models and mechanisms in renal disease, in Schrier R.W. (ed.): *Renal and Electrolyte Disorders.* Boston, Little, Brown & Co., 1976, p. 423. Used by permission.)

tive, sclerosing, or membranous features. According to traditional concepts, immune-complex glomerulonephritis results from the formation of soluble antibody-antigen complexes in the circulation and their subsequent deposition in glomeruli. The site of immune-complex deposition and the type of glomerular damage induced has been attributed to a number of factors, including the amount of antigen entering the circulation, the intensity of the antibody response, and the composition and size of the immune-complexes.

Animal models of acute and chronic serum sickness have served as prototypes of immune-complex glomerulonephritis. In experimental serum sickness, circulating immune-complexes are generated by one or more injections of heterologous serum or heterologous plasma proteins. Studies of serum sickness models suggest that the proclivity of circulating immune-complexes to produce glomerular injury depends on the size of the antibody-antigen complex (Fig 2–7). In the presence of either antibody or antigen excess, small immune-complexes are formed and presumably escape entrapment within the glomerular capillaries. Small complexes tend not to be pathogenic since they are incapable of fixing complement. By contrast, very large immune-complexes may form when antibody and antigen are present in equivalent amounts, because antibody molecules can form bridges between antigens (see Fig 2–7). Large antibody-antigen complexes are rapidly cleared from the circulation by the reticuloendothelial system and rarely lead to glomerular injury. In experimental serum sickness, pathogenic immune-complexes are usually intermediate in size and tend to form in the presence of a slight antigen excess or slight antibody excess. Among the intermediate-sized nephritogenic complexes, size also determines where the complexes will become localized. Larger complexes are most likely taken up by phagocytic mesangial cells, while smaller complexes may pass through the mesangium to be trapped in the glomerular basement membrane.

These traditional concepts regarding the pathogenesis of immune-complex glomerulonephritis have been challenged by the recent discovery that some glomerular immune-deposits may result not from deposition of circulating immune-complexes, but from formation in situ of immune-complexes resulting from the reaction of circulating antibodies to free antigens previously fixed within the glomerular capillary wall.[39, 40] When chronic serum sickness is induced by injections of cationic bovine serum albumin, the free antigen localizes in the glomerulus prior to an antibody response. In this and other experimental models of in situ immune-complex glomerulonephritis, immune-deposits tend to form in the subepithelial portion of the glomerular basement membrane (Fig 2–8). The development of subepithelial deposits appears to be dependent on the charge of the antigen and independent of the strength of the antibody response or the size of the circulating immune-complexes.[41] Highly cationic antigens of appropriate size penetrate the capillary wall and concentrate in the

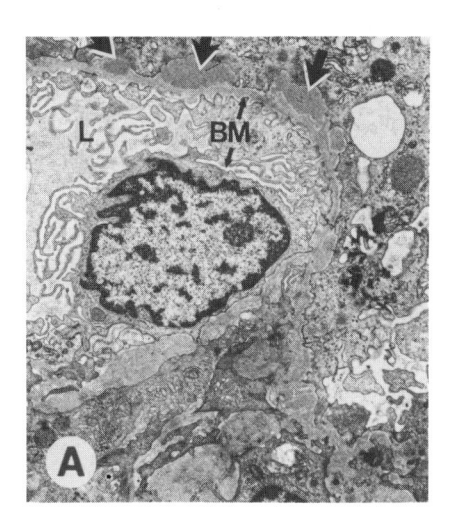

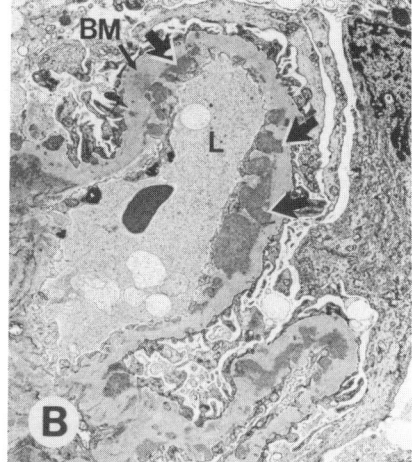

Fig 2–8.—Location of basement membrane deposits in immune-complex glomerulonephritis. **A,** subepithelial deposits *(large arrows)* in post-infectious glomerulonephritis; ×13,100. **B,** subendothelial deposits *(large arrows)* in lupus nephritis; ×5,400. L = capillary lumen; BM = basement membrane.

subepithelial space due to charge interactions with fixed anionic sites. The free antigens subsequently induce an antibody response resulting in immune-deposit formation. This theory of immune-complex formation is consistent with earlier observations that antigen excess favors the development of glomerular injury, since the presence of excess antigen would allow for the initial deposition of free antigen within the glomerular basement membrane.

In contrast to the subepithelial location of immune-deposits induced by an in situ mechanism, infusions of preformed immune-complexes usually produce only mesangial or occasionally subendothelial deposits (see Fig 2–8). Whereas in situ formation of subepithelial deposits has been clearly correlated with the development of proteinuria, there is actually little direct evidence that mesangial trapping of circulating immune-complexes initiates glomerular injury or proteinuria. Nevertheless, proteinuria is clinically observed in a number of human glomerulopathies characterized by mesangial or subendothelial immune-deposits. The exact mechanisms of immune-complex formation, the factors determining the site of glomerular immune-cómplex localization, and the mechanisms by which immune-deposits induce proteinuria remain to be fully elucidated. Although glomerular immune-deposits may directly alter the structure of the glomerular capillary wall, in most cases these deposits are inciting agents that evoke a variety of secondary inflammatory responses that are more directly responsible for inducing proteinuria.

Inflammatory Mediators of Immunologically Induced Proteinuria

Proteinuria due to glomerular antibody deposition generally requires the activation of some additional mediator system. In certain experimental models of antiglomerular basement membrane disease, antibody deposition alone may alter the functional and structural integrity of the basement membrane sufficiently to produce proteinuria in the absence of secondary immune reactants. In this section we review those secondary inflammatory responses that more typically mediate proteinuria following the deposition of immune-deposits.

Complement and Neutrophils

The role of complement and neutrophils in mediating proteinuria has been studied most extensively in the heterologous phase of nephrotoxic serum nephritis, an experimental model of antiglomerular basement membrane disease. In this model, the deposition of antiglomerular basement membrane antibody is accompanied by complement activation, deposition of C3 within the basement membrane, and the development of a glomerular cellular infiltrate composed of mononuclear cells and neutrophils.[42] Complement fixation promotes the immune adherence of neutrophils via C3b receptors and also generates soluble products of the complement cascade, such as C3a and C5a, which act as chemotaxins and stimulate the release of hydrolytic enzymes by neutrophils. The neutrophil dependency of proteinuria in this model has been demonstrated by studies in which prior neutrophil depletion by specific antineutrophil antibodies or nitrogen mustard abolishes the proteinuria.[43, 44] Neutrophils may alter glomerular permselectivity in a number of ways. Lysosomal enzymes released by leukocytes may directly hydrolyze the glomerular basement membrane. In addition, a number of peptides contained within lysozomes are vasoactive substances that may directly alter the permeability of the glomerular capillary membrane. In neutrophil-dependent models of glomerular injury, proteinuria tends to be nonselective, suggesting that hydrolytic enzymes released by leukocytes may directly increase the size of pores within the basement membrane. However, alterations in the charge-selective properties of the glomerulus may also play a role in mediating proteinuria, as suggested by a reduction in glomerular polyanion content in these models.[45]

An effect of the complement system in independently mediating proteinuria has been demonstrated in experimental models of in situ immune-complex glomerular disease manifested by subepithelial deposits.[32] This pattern of immune-deposit formation can be induced by antibodies reacting with exogenous cationic antigens previously fixed within the basement membrane,[41] or by antibodies reacting with a fixed glomerular antigen in a subepithelial location.[46] The histologic appearance of the glomerulus in these experimental models resembles human membranous nephropathy and is notable for the absence of cellular poliferation. The development of subepithelial deposits and the onset of proteinuria are accompanied by deposition of C3 within the basement membrane. Depletion of complement by prior administration of cobra venom factor abolishes the proteinuria in these models,[34] suggesting that complement directly alters glomerular permselectivity. Although activation of the complement system may generate a number of chemotaxins, the absence of a cellular infiltrate in experimental models of membranous nephropathy suggests that the proteinuria is not dependent on the presence of inflammatory cells. Indeed, selective neutrophil depletion by antineutrophil antibodies has no effect on the onset or magnitude of proteinuria in these models. The exact mechanisms of complement-induced proteinuria have not been fully defined. It is of interest that the onset of proteinuria in models of membranous nephropathy is not initially associated with a reduction in glomerular polyanion content,[47] suggesting that proteinuria does not result from an alteration in the electrostatic charge of the capillary membrane. It has been postulated that the terminal components of the complement cascade may exert a direct membranolytic effect—a process that may be analogous to complement-mediated red blood cell lysis, and which presumably increases the effective pore size of the glomerular basement membrane.

Other Possible Mediators of Glomerular Injury and Proteinuria

A possible role for the coagulation system in the pathogenesis of glomerulonephritis is supported by the finding of glomerular fibrin and related proteins in a variety of experimental and clinical forms of glomerular disease. However, there is little evidence that components of the coagulation system directly cause proteinuria.

It has been postulated that platelets may play a role in the pathogenesis of certain glomerular diseases since they provide a source of vasoactive amines (e.g., serotonin, histamine) as well as the vasoconstrictor prostaglandin, thromboxane. Although such vasoactive substances may modify urinary protein excretion by altering glomerular hemodynamics, there is no evidence that they directly alter glomerular permselectivity. The effects of other renal vasoactive hormones (e.g., the renin-angiotensin system, prostaglandins, and the kallikrein-kinin system) on glomerular permselectivity remain to be elucidated.

Cell-Mediated Mechanisms of Glomerular Injury

Cell-mediated immune mechanisms have been implicated in the pathogenesis of certain interstitial renal diseases; however, recent evidence suggests that cell-mediated mechanisms may also initiate or perpetuate glomerular injury. Speculation has centered on the possibility that a soluble product of sensitized lymphocytes may directly alter glomerular permeability in patients with minimal change nephropathy.[32] This hypothesis is supported by recent studies in rats that demonstrate a reduction in glomerular charge following the infusion of supernatants from cultured lymphocytes of patients with nephrotic syndrome.[33] In addition to the possible role of lymphokines in initiating glomerular injury, indirect evidence suggests that antibody-directed, delayed hypersensitivity reactions may contribute to glomerular injury. Mononuclear cells, in the form of macrophages, are important mediators of glomerular injury in a number of models of glomerulonephritis.[48] Furthermore, selective macrophage depletion induced by specific antimacrophage serum completely abolishes proteinuria in some of these models.[49] Macrophages and lymphocytes bearing Fc receptors may be directed to induce glomerular injury by antibodies bound within the glomerular capillary wall. Macrophage recruitment could also be directed by lymphokines released by sensitized T-cells responding to glomerular antigens. It is difficult to separate the effects of these cellular mechanisms from those of antibody deposition, complement activation, and/or neutrophil recruitment which generally induce capillary wall injury and proteinuria long before the onset of delayed hypersensitivity.

MECHANISMS OF FUNCTIONAL PROTEINURIA

The common causes of functional proteinuria, i.e., proteinuria occurring in the absence of renal parenchymal disease, are outlined in Chapter 1. The pathophysiology of functional proteinuria is incompletely understood. Most of the conditions associated with functional proteinuria are accompanied by renal vasoconstriction, suggesting a hemodynamic basis for this phenomenon. In many clinical circumstances, modest reductions in renal blood flow are accompanied by a variety of neurogenic and humoral reactions that preserve the glomerular filtration rate. This autoregulation of glomerular filtration rate in the presence of reduced renal plasma flow increases the filtration fraction (i.e., the ratio of glomerular filtration rate to renal plasma flow). As the filtration fraction rises, the concentration of plasma proteins progressively increases toward the efferent end of the glomerular capillary (Fig 2–9). Because the glomerular capillary membrane is relatively, but not absolutely, impermeable to circulating macromolecules, this increment in the concentration gradient for plasma proteins across the capillary wall favors the movement of weakly permeant proteins into the proximal nephron.

Whether this mechanism fully accounts for all forms of functional proteinuria remains a matter of speculation. The filtration fraction is usually increased during exercise[50, 51] and in patients with congestive heart failure, but there is little data available regarding alterations

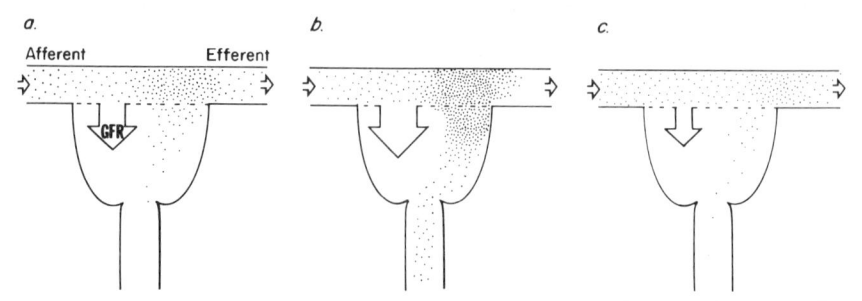

Fig 2–9.—Influence of filtration fraction on urinary protein excretion. *a*, under normal conditions, glomerular ultrafiltration results in a gradual increment in the concentration of protein toward the efferent end of the capillary, and small amounts of protein leak into the urine. *b*, increased filtration fraction magnifies the concentration of protein in the efferent capillary, and urinary protein excretion increases. *c*, reduced filtration fraction reduces efferent capillary protein concentration, and urinary protein excretion declines.

in the filtration fraction of patients with other conditions associated with functional proteinuria. A recent study has demonstrated that fractional dextran clearances are increased in patients with cardiac failure.[52] However, the same study also showed that the fractional clearance of albumin was disproportionately greater than the enhanced clearance of comparably sized neutral dextrans,[52] suggesting that alterations in glomerular electrostatic barrier function or in the tubular handling of albumin may compound the effects of an increased filtration fraction in mediating proteinuria associated with cardiac failure. Similarly, studies of exercising dogs have demonstrated an almost 50% decrease in colloidal iron staining of the glomerular capillary membrane,[53] a phenomenon suggesting that alterations in glomerular charge may play a role in exercise-induced proteinuria. It remains to be proved whether similar mechanisms are operative in other forms of functional proteinuria.

REFERENCES

1. Oken D.E., Flamenbaum W.: Micropuncture studies of proximal tubule albumin concentrations in normal and nephrotic rats. *J. Clin. Invest.* 50:1498, 1971.
2. Maunsbauch A.B.: Absorption of I^{125}-labeled homologous albumin by rat kidney proximal tubule cells. *J. Ultrastruct. Res.* 15:197, 1966.
3. Carone F.A., Peterson D.R., Fluret G.: Renal tubular handling of small peptide hormones. *J. Lab. Clin. Med.* 100:1, 1982.
4. Bohrer M.P., Deen W.M., Robertson C.R., et al.: Mechanisms of angiotensin II-induced proteinuria in the rat. *Am. J. Physiol.* 233:F13, 1977.
5. Chang R.L.S., Robertson C.R., Deen W.M., et al.: Permselectivity of the glomerular capillary wall to macromolecules: I. Theoretical considerations. *Biophys. J.* 15:861, 1975.

6. Brenner B.M., Bohrer M.P., Baylis C., et al.: Determinations of glomerular permselectivity: insights derived from observations in vivo. *Kidney Int.* 12:229, 1977.
7. Pappenheimer J.R.: Passage of molecules through capillary walls. *Physiol. Rev.* 33:387, 1953.
8. Farquar M.G., Wissig S.L., Palade G.E.: Glomerular permeability: I. Ferritin transfer across the normal glomerular capillary walls. *J. Exp. Med.* 113:47, 1961.
9. Graham R.C., Karnovsky M.J.: Glomerular permeability: ultrastructural and cytochemical studies using peroxidases as protein tracers. *J. Exp. Med.* 124:1123, 1966.
10. Graham R.C., Kellermeyer R.W.: Bovine lactoperoxidases as a cytochemical protein tracer for electron microscopy. *J. Histochem. Cytochem.* 16:275, 1968.
11. Venkatachalam M.A., Karnovsky M.J., Fahimi H.D., et al.: An ultrastructural study of glomerular permeability using catalase and peroxidase as tracer proteins. *J. Exp. Med.* 132:1153, 1970.
12. Ryan G.B., Karnovsky M.J.: Distribution of endogenous albumin in the rat glomerulus: Role of hemodynamic factors in glomerular barrier function. *Kidney Int.* 9:36, 1976.
13. Bennet C.M., Glassock R.J., Chang R.L.S., et al.: Permselectivity of the glomerular capillary wall: studies of experimental glomerulonephritis in the rat using dextran sulfate. *J. Clin. Invest.* 57:1287, 1976.
14. Bohrer M.P., Baylis C., Humes H.D., et al.: Permselectivity of the glomerular capillary wall: facilitated filtration of circulating polycations. *J. Clin. Invest.* 61:72, 1978.
15. Rennke H.G., Venkatachalam M.A.: Glomerular permeability: in vivo tracer studies with polyanionic and polycationic ferritins. *Kidney Int.* 11:44, 1977.
16. Rennke H.G., Cotran R.S., Venkatachalam M.A.: Role of molecular charge in glomerular permeability: tracer studies with cationized ferritins. *J. Cell Biol.* 67:638, 1975.
17. Kanwar Y.S., Farguar J.G.: Presence of heparan sulfate in the glomerular basement membrane. *Proc. Natl. Acad. Sci. U.S.A.* 76:1303, 1979.
18. Kanwar Y.S., Hascall V.C., Farguar M.G.: Partial characterization of newly synthesized proteoglycans isolated from the glomerular basement membrane. *J. Cell Biol.* 90:527, 1981.
19. Vernier R.L., Klein D.J., Sisson S.P., et al.: Heparan sulfate-rich anionic sites in the human glomerular basement membrane. *N. Engl. J. Med.* 309:1001, 1983.
20. Kanwar Y.S., Linker A., Farguar M.G.: Increased permeability of the glomerular basement membrane to ferritin after removal of glycosamino-glycans (heparan sulfate) by enzyme digestion. *J. Cell. Biol.* 86:688, 1980.
21. Rosenzweig L.J., Kanwar Y.S.: Removal of sulfated (heparan sulfate) or nonsulfated (hyaluronic acid) glycosaminglycans results in increased permeability of the glomerular basement membrane to ^{125}I bovine serum albumin. *Lab. Invest.* 47:177, 1982.
22. Harrison J.F., Lunt G.S., Scott P., et al.: Urinary lysozyme, ribonuclease, and low-molecular-weight protein in renal disease. *Lancet* 1:371, 1968.
23. Osserman E.F., Lawlor D.P.: Serum and urinary lysozyme (murmidase) in monomyelocytic leukemia. *J. Exp. Med.* 124:921, 1966.
24. Chang R.L.S., Deen W.M., Robertson C.R., et al.: Permselectivity of the glomerular capillary wall: Studies of experimental glomerulonephritis in the rat using neutral dextran. *J. Clin. Invest.* 57:1272, 1976.
25. Bohere M.P., Baylis C., Robertson C.R., et al.: Mechanisms of puromycin-induced defects in the trans-glomerular passage of water and macromolecules. *J. Clin. Invest.* 60:152, 1977.
26. Michael A.F., Blau E.B., Vernier R.L.: Glomerular polyanion: alteration in aminonucleoside nephrosis. *Lab. Invest.* 23:649, 1970.
27. Blau E.B., Haas D.E.: Glomerular sialic acid and proteinuria in human renal disease. *Lab. Invest.* 28:477, 1973.

28. Winetz J.A., Robertson C.R., Colbetz H.V., et al.: The nature of the glomerular injury in minimal change and focal sclerosing glomerulopathies. *Am. J. Kidney Dis.* 1:91, 1981.
29. Myers B.D., Winetz J.A., Chui F., et al.: Mechanisms of proteinuria in diabetic nephropathy. *Kidney Int.* 21:633–641, 1982.
30. Shalhoub R.J.: Pathogenesis of lipoid nephrosis: A disorder of T-cell function. *Lancet* 2:556, 1974.
31. Boulton Jones J.M., Tulloch I., Dore B., et al.: Changes in the glomerular capillary wall induced by lymphocyte products and serum of nephrotic patients. *Clin. Nephrol.* 20:72, 1983.
32. Salant D.J., Belok S., Madaio M.P., et al.: A new role for complement in experimental membranous nephropathy in rats. *J. Clin. Invest.* 66:1339, 1980.
33. Deen W.M., Maddox D.A., Robertson C.R., et al.: Dynamics of glomerular ultrafiltration in the rat: VII. Response to reduced renal mass. *Am. J. Physiol.* 227:556, 1974.
34. Eisenbach G.M., VanLiew J.B., Boylan J.W.: Effect of angiotensin on the filtration of protein in the rat kidney: a micropuncture study. *Kidney Int.* 8:80, 1975.
35. Robson A.M., Mor J., Root E.R., et al.: Mechanism of proteinuria in nonglomerular renal disease. *Kidney Int.* 16:426, 1979.
36. Brenner B.M., Hostetter T.H., Humes H.D.: Molecular basis of proteinuria of glomerular origin. *N. Engl. J. Med.* 298:826, 1978.
37. Bhathena D.B., Weiss J.H., Holland N.H., et al.: Focal and segmental glomerular sclerosis in reflux nephropathy. *Am. J. Med.* 68:886, 1980.
38. Couser W.B., Salant O.J.: Immunopathogenesis of glomerular capillary wall injury in nephrotic states, in Brenner B.M., Stein J.H. (eds.): *Contemporary Issues in Nephrology,* Volume 9. New York, Churchill, Livingstone, Inc., 1982, vol. 4, p. 48.
39. Van Es L.A., Blok A.P.R., Schenfield L., et al.: Chronic nephritis induced by antibodies reacting with glomerular-bound immune complexes. *Kidney Int.* 11:106, 1977.
40. Couser W.G., Salant D.J.: In situ immune complex formation and glomerular injury. *Kidney Int.* 17:1, 1980.
41. Adler S.G., Wang H., Ward H.J., et al.: Electrical charge. Its role in the pathogenesis and prevention of experimental membranous nephropathy in the rabbit. *J. Clin. Invest.* 71:487, 1983.
42. Shigematsu H.: Glomerular events during the initial phase of rat Masugi nephritis. *Virchows Archiv.* 5:187, 1970.
43. Cochrane C.G., Unanue E., Dixon F.J.: A role of polymorphonuclear leukocytes and complement in nephrotoxic nephritis. *J. Exp. Med.* 122:99, 1965.
44. Hawkins D., Cochrane C.G.: Glomerular basement membrane damage in immunological glomerular nephritis. *Immunology* 14:665, 1968.
45. Kreisberg J.I., Wayne D.B., Karnovsky M.J.: Rapid and focal loss of negative charge associated with mononuclear cell infiltration early in nephrotoxic serum nephritis. *Kidney Int.* 16:290, 1979.
46. Couser W.G., Steinmuller D.S., Stilmant M.M., et al.: Experimental glomerulonephritis in the isolated perfused rat kidney. *J. Clin. Invest.* 62:1275, 1978.
47. Couser W.G., Silmant M.M., Darby C.: Autologous immune complex nephropathy: I. Sequential study of immune complex deposition, ultrastructural changes, proteinuria and alterations in glomerular sialoproteins. *Lab. Invest.* 34:23, 1976.
48. Holdsworth S.R., Neale T.J., Wilson C.B.: The participation of macrophages and monocytes in experimental immune complex glomerulonephritis. *Clin. Immunol. Immunopathol.* 15:1510, 1980.
49. Holdsworth S.R., Neale T.J., Wilson C.B.: Abrogation of macrophage dependent injury in experimental glomerulonephritis in the rabbit. Use of an anti-macrophage serum. *J. Clin. Invest.* 68:686, 1981.
50. Grimby G.: Renal clearances during prolonged supine exercises at different loads. *J. Appl. Physiol.* 20:1294, 1965.

51. Poortsman J.R.: Postexercise proteinuria in humans. *J.A.M.A.* 253:236, 1985.
52. Carrie B., Hilberman M., Schroeder J., et al.: Albuminuria and the permselective properties of the glomerulus in cardiac failure. *Kidney Int.* 17:507, 1980.
53. Zambraski E.J., Bober M.C., Goldstein J.E., et al.: Changes in renal cortical sialic acids and colloidal iron staining associated with exercise. *Med. Sci. Sports Exerc.* 13:229, 1981.

3 The Nephrotic Syndrome: Consequences of Heavy Proteinuria

HEAVY PROTEINURIA OCCURS almost exclusively among patients with renal diseases that primarily affect the glomeruli. In adults, a urinary protein excretion rate greater than 3.0 gm per day virtually assures the presence of an underlying glomerulopathy. Protein excretion of this magnitude is frequently accompanied by a constellation of clinical and laboratory abnormalities collectively referred to as the nephrotic syndrome. Hypoalbuminemia, edema, hyperlipidemia, and lipiduria are the most consistently observed features of this syndrome. Because these clinical abnormalities represent physiologic consequences of heavy proteinuria, their presence and severity vary depending on the magnitude of urinary protein losses. This variability in clinical manifestations makes precise diagnostic criteria for the nephrotic syndrome difficult to formulate. The definition of nephrotic syndrome rests fundamentally on the demonstration of proteinuria of sufficient magnitude to be accounted for by glomerular disease. Secondary manifestations such as hypoalbuminemia, edema, and hyperlipidemia serve to corroborate the clinical suspicion of an underlying glomerulopathy, and generally correlate well with the degree of proteinuria. Although protein excretion rates greater than 3.0 gm per day bring attention to glomerular disease, the designation of "nephrotic" and "non-nephrotic" proteinuria based on such quantitative criteria should not be overemphasized because most of the glomerulopathies that cause the nephrotic syndrome can be associated with mild, asymptomatic proteinuria.

Once regarded as a single disease entity, the nephrotic syndrome is now recognized as the common manifestation of a variety of disease processes, each characterized by increased permeability of the glomerular capillary wall to circulating plasma proteins. The nephrotic syndrome occurs secondary to a broad spectrum of pathologic states including certain infectious diseases, neoplasms, drugs, toxins, and multisystem and heredofamilial disorders. Another group of cases classified as the idiopathic nephrotic syndrome, by definition, occurs in the absence of an obvious cause. The underlying diseases associated with nephrotic syndrome are discussed in greater detail in Chapters 4 and 5. In this chapter, we focus on the expected physiologic consequences and potential complications of heavy proteinuria.

COMMON CONSEQUENCES OF HEAVY PROTEINURIA

Hypoalbuminemia

In general, hypoalbuminemia may result from urinary protein loss, gastrointestinal protein loss, reduced dietary protein intake, reduced hepatic protein synthesis, increased protein catabolism, or changes in the internal distribution of the body's albumin pool. In patients with nephrotic syndrome, some or all of these factors may be present. Patients with heavy proteinuria usually manifest some degree of hypoalbuminemia (less than 3.0 gm/dl); however, the relationship between the magnitude of proteinuria and hypoalbuminemia is quite variable. Malnourished elderly patients or patients with liver disease may develop profound hypoalbuminemia with relatively moderate urinary protein losses, whereas young, otherwise healthy patients may excrete considerably more than 3.0 gm of protein per day without developing notable hypoalbuminemia.

Urinary losses of albumin and the catabolism of excessive amounts of filtered albumin by the renal tubules are the most important pathogenetic factors accounting for hypoalbuminemia in the nephrotic syndrome. Loss of protein in the urine is clearly not the sole factor accounting for hypoalbuminemia since hepatic albumin synthesis should be able to compensate for urinary albumin losses. In normal adults, albumin synthetic and catabolic rates are about 10 to 16 gm per day, reflecting a daily turnover of 5% to 10% of the intravascular albumin pool. In patients with the nephrotic syndrome, turnover studies employing radiolabeled albumin have shown that hepatic synthesis of albumin may increase two to five times above normal (i.e., 20 to 80 gm per day) in the absence of coexisting liver disease or malnutrition.[1,2] Since the urinary loss of protein in nephrotic subjects is usually considerably less than these amounts (ranging from 3 to 30 gm per day), urinary loss of albumin does not by itself account for hypoalbuminemia in most cases.

Under normal circumstances, 40% of the total body albumin pool is distributed in the intravascular space with the remaining 60% present in extravascular compartments. In the absence of a glomerular protein leak, the liver and gastrointestinal tract constitute the primary sites for albumin catabolism. Patients with the nephrotic syndrome have a markedly reduced total albumin pool, with a change in the distribution of albumin such that a greater fraction of the total pool is intravascular.[1] Because nephrotic patients have a reduced albumin pool, their absolute rate of albumin catabolism may be below normal. However, the fractional catabolism of albumin (i.e., the amount of albumin catabolized/total albumin pool) is usually increased and plays an important role in the maintenance of hypoalbuminemia. There are conflicting data regarding the role of the gastrointestinal tract in this enhanced catabolism of albumin, but the kidney itself appears to be the major site of increased albumin catabolism in the nephrotic syndrome. The normal kidney usually accounts for no more than 10% of total albumin catabolism. In the nephrotic syndrome, enhanced glomerular permeability results in the filtration of large quantities of albumin that are subject to proximal tubular reabsorption and degradation. Clearance studies in humans with the nephrotic syndrome demonstrate that the amount of albumin filtered across the glomerular capillary membrane may exceed 50 gm per day.[3] As indicated above, daily urinary protein excretion in nephrotic subjects is usually much less than this, suggesting that a considerable fraction of filtered albumin is catabolized by the renal tubules. The catabolic rate for albumin increases with increasing proteinuria, indicating that tubular reabsorption and degradation increase as the nephrotic condition worsens.[4,5] Evidence from animal models of nephrotic syndrome suggests that the kidney may account for 50% of total albumin catabolism in the presence of heavy proteinuria.[6]

The combined effects of urinary albumin loss and increased albumin catabolism in the nephrotic syndrome are apparently sufficient to overcome any compensatory increase in hepatic albumin synthesis and usually result in some degree of hypoalbuminemia in patients with heavy proteinuria. Furthermore, continued urinary protein losses may ultimately deplete substrate for protein synthesis by the liver, leading to a relative reduction in the rate of hepatic albumin synthesis. Although there is no precise quantitative relationship between the magnitude of proteinuria and hypoalbuminemia, it is generally true that the greater the urinary protein excretion, the lower

```
┌─────────────────────────────────────────────────────────┐
│ INCREASED GLOMERULAR PERMEABILITY TO PLASMA PROTEINS    │
└─────────────────────────────────────────────────────────┘
         ↙                ⇓                    
  ┌───────────┐      ┌──────────┐    ┌────────────────────┐
  │ALBUMINURIA│      │ LIPIDURIA│◄───│HYPERLIPOPROTEINEMIA│
  └───────────┘      └──────────┘    └────────────────────┘
      ↙                                        ⇑
┌──────────────────┐              ┌────────────────────────┐
│TUBULAR CATABOLISM│              │ INCREASED HEPATIC SYNTHESIS │
│OF FILTERED ALBUMIN│             │ OF ALBUMIN, LIPOPROTEINS │
└──────────────────┘              └────────────────────────┘
      ⇓                                        ⇑
┌────────────────┐          ┌──────────────────────────────┐
│HYPOALBUMINEMIA │─────────►│DECREASED PLASMA ONCOTIC PRESSURE│
└────────────────┘          └──────────────────────────────┘
                                           ⇓
                         ┌────────────────────────────┐
                         │DECREASED INTRAVASCULAR VOLUME│
                         └────────────────────────────┘
                                           ⇓
                       ┌──────────────────────────────────┐
                       │RENAL RETENTION OF SODIUM AND WATER│
                       └──────────────────────────────────┘
                                           ⇓
                                      ┌───────┐
                                      │ EDEMA │
                                      └───────┘
```

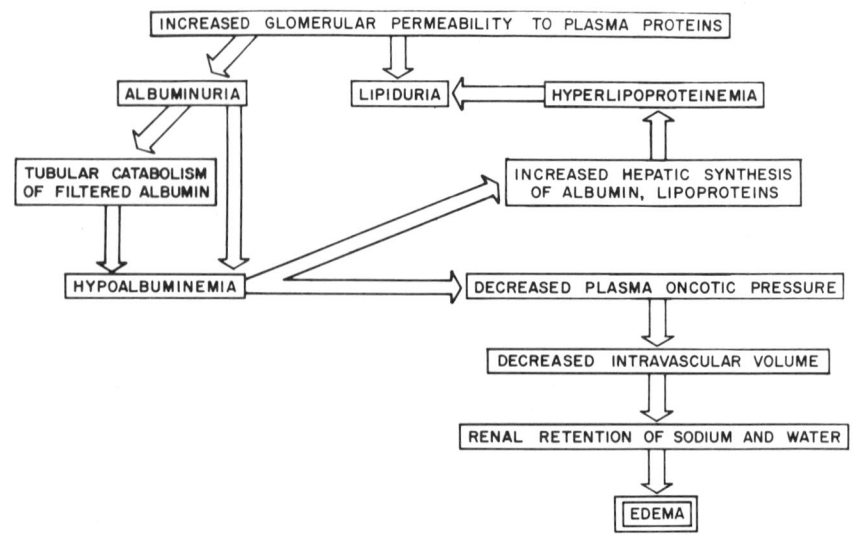

Fig 3–1.—Consequences of heavy proteinuria resulting from increased glomerular permeability to plasma proteins.

the serum albumin concentration. Hypoalbuminemia, in turn, plays a pivotal pathophysiologic role in the development of other common features of the nephrotic syndrome (Fig 3–1).

Edema

Generalized edema is the most common presenting symptom of patients with heavy proteinuria, but the mechanisms of edema formation in the nephrotic syndrome are not entirely understood. Edema represents an accumulation of interstitial fluid resulting from a disturbance in one of the critical capillary Starling forces that influence extracellular fluid distribution between the intravascular and interstitial compartments. These Starling forces can be expressed in the following equation:

$$V = K_f[(P_c - P_i) - \sigma(\pi_c - \pi_i)]$$

where V is the net volume flow from the intravascular to the interstitial compartment, K_f is the permeability coefficient of the capillary membrane, P_c is the intracapillary hydrostatic pressure, P_i is the interstitial hydrostatic pressure, σ is the reflection coefficient for plasma protein, and π_c and π_i are the oncotic pressures of the plasma and interstitial fluid, respectively. Under normal circumstances, the net hydrostatic pressure gradient (P_c-P_i) slightly exceeds the net oncotic pressure gradient (π_c-π_i), so that small amounts of water move from the intravascular to the interstitial space. This interstitial water is returned to the circulation via the lymphatics. In accordance with these concepts, edema may develop when the hydrostatic pressure gradient across the capillary membrane increases, when the oncotic pressure gradient decreases, when lymphatic flow is obstructed, or when the inherent permeability of the capillary membrane is increased.

Traditional teaching suggests that, in the nephrotic syndrome, edema forms because hypoalbuminemia reduces plasma oncotic pressure and shifts capillary forces toward greater filtration into tissue spaces. Although plasma oncotic pressure is reduced throughout the intravascular compartment, patients with the nephrotic syndrome typically develop edema in locations where capillary hydrostatic pressure is highest (e.g., dependent areas) and where interstitial hydrostatic pressure is lowest (e.g., scrotal, periorbital, and facial tissues). Fluid accumulates in the interstitial compartment until a new steady state is achieved in which increased interstitial pressure balances the net reduction in plasma oncotic pressure. This redistribution of extracellular fluid presumably reduces intravascular volume and evokes a variety of homeostatic mechanisms, including stimulation of the renin-aldosterone axis, release of antidiuretic hormone from the hypothalamus, and possibly inhibition of a natriuretic hormone. These perturbations signal the kidney to retain sodium and water. Retention of fluid, in turn, serves to replenish the intravascular volume, but this fluid accumulation is counterproductive because it expands the extracellular volume further, dilutes available plasma proteins, and yields more edema. This traditional explanation for the pathogenesis of edema in the nephrotic syndrome differs significantly from the mechanisms operative in other edematous disorders such as congestive heart failure and cirrhosis. In the latter disorders, renal sodium retention initiates extracellular volume expansion and thereby causes edema. In the nephrotic syndrome, this relationship is reversed so that edema formation is the cause, rather than the effect, of renal sodium retention.

The above theory of sodium accumulation in the nephrotic syndrome would predict the presence of decreased plasma volume and elevated plasma renin and aldosterone levels secondary to hypovolemia. Two lines of evidence suggest that this conventional view of the pathogenesis of edema may not be entirely correct, or at least might not be valid for all cases of nephrotic syndrome. First is the paradoxical absence of edema in many patients with congenital analbuminemia, a finding which suggests that hypoalbuminemia may not be the sole determinant of edema formation in the nephrotic syndrome. Subtle differences between these two conditions may account for the absence of edema in congenital analbuminemia, however. Compared to analbuminemic patients, patients with the nephrotic syndrome may sustain greater reductions in plasma oncotic pressure resulting from the excretion of plasma proteins other than albumin. Patients with analbuminemia may exhibit a compensatory reduction in capillary hydrostatic pressure or an increased rate of lymphatic flow that may completely offset the reduction in plasma oncotic pressure and thus prevent accumulation of fluid within the interstitial compartment.[7] The kidneys of patients with analbuminemia may have an increased ability to excrete a salt load.[8] Finally, it has been postulated that patients with nephrotic syndrome, unlike patients with analbuminemia, may have a diffuse capillary defect resulting in increased capillary permeability in both the glomeruli and in the extrarenal vasculature. The second line of conflicting evidence regarding the pathogenesis of nephrotic edema comes from studies demonstrating normal or increased plasma volumes and suppressed renin and aldosterone levels in some patients with the nephrotic syndrome.[9, 10] Renin-sodium profiles have confirmed the existence of a subset of nephrotic patients who are hypervolemic and who have low plasma renin and aldosterone concentrations that return toward normal after sodium depletion.[10] These patients usually have overt structural glomerular damage and commonly have hypertension and moderate reductions in glomerular filtration rate, observations that raise the possibility that the reduction in glomerular filtration rate may account for the impaired ability to excrete sodium. These clinical observations suggest that nephrotic patients are heterogeneous with respect to their plasma volume status and that the mechanisms of edema formation may vary depending on the underlying glomerular histopathology.

The kidney's role in the genesis of positive sodium balance in the nephrotic syndrome is not fully understood. In the absence of advanced renal parenchymal disease, glomerular filtration rate may be increased, normal, or decreased. The filtration fraction (i.e., the ratio of glomerular filtration rate to renal plasma flow) is variable among nephrotic subjects and may be inversely related to plasma volume.[9] In most animal models of nephrotic syndrome, filtration fraction is decreased. In experimental nephrotic syndrome in the rat, direct micropuncture of superficial proximal nephrons demonstrates that absolute proximal tubular sodium reabsorption is decreased, a finding consistent with the predicted effects of a low filtration fraction on peritubular Starling forces.[11] The depressed proximal tubular reabsorption implies that delivery of tubular fluid to the distal tubule is enhanced. The distal nephron thus appears to be responsible for the renal sodium retention characteristic of the nephrotic syndrome. Although aldosterone clearly accelerates the rate of distal tubular sodium reabsorption, it is unlikely that increased distal sodium reabsorption results solely from secondary hyperaldosteronism since nephrotic patients with expanded plasma volumes and suppressed aldosterone levels continue to retain sodium.[10] Other causes of increased sodium reabsorption in the distal tubule of nephrotic patients remain to be defined. Theoretically, renal sodium retention could result from redistribution of renal blood flow from superficial to deep cortical nephrons that have a higher inherent capacity for sodium reabsorption; however, this hypothesis has not been fully explored in experimental models of nephrotic syndrome. Similarly, it is possible that nephrotic patients fail to elaborate a natriuretic hormone, but the very existence of such a hormone remains speculative. Although many questions remain unanswered regarding the mechanisms of renal sodium retention in the nephrotic syndrome, it is clear that the kidney plays a central role in maintaining positive sodium balance in patients with heavy proteinuria.

Hyperlipidemia and Lipiduria

The presence of hyperlipidemia is not essential for the diagnosis of nephrotic syndrome, but an increase in the concentration of plasma lipids is often a striking finding associated with heavy proteinuria. In general, an increase in plasma lipids may result from an increase in their rate of synthesis or a decrease in their rate of catabolism. Both factors play a role in the development of hyperlipidemia in the nephrotic syndrome.

In most studies of nephrotic subjects, the serum albumin concentration is inversely related to elevations in plasma concentrations of cholesterol and phospholipids. The observation that lipids exist in plasma as lipoproteins has helped to explain the pathogenesis of hyperlipidemia in the nephrotic syndrome. Albumin and very low density lipoproteins (VLDL) share common synthetic and secretory pathways in the hepatocyte. Increased synthesis of albumin by the hepatocyte in response to hypoalbuminemia may inadvertently stimulate the synthesis of lipid apoproteins and VLDL.[12] Thus, lipoproteins are "innocent bystanders" in a homeostatic reaction that is designed to increase albumin production. Compatible with this hypothesis are studies that demonstrate a transient reduction in plasma lipid concentrations when nephrotic subjects are infused with albumin.[13] In nephrotic rats, serum lipid levels decline following the administration of albumin, dextran, polyvinylpyrrolidone or gamma globulin, suggesting that changes in colloid osmotic pressure or plasma volume, rather than the concentration of albumin per se, regulate hepatic albumin and lipoprotein synthesis.[14] Although patients with analbuminemia develop a serum lipid profile similar to that of nephrotic patients, hyperlipidemia does not routinely occur in other conditions associated with hypoalbuminemia, such as cirrhosis, malnutrition, or the protein-losing enteropathies. These latter conditions are not analogous to the nephrotic syndrome, however, because reduced hepatic synthetic capacity or lack of nutritional substrate accounts both for hypoalbuminemia and the absence of excessive lipoprotein synthesis.

Normal lipoprotein metabolic pathways are shown schematically in Figure 3–2. Under normal circumstances, VLDL produced by the

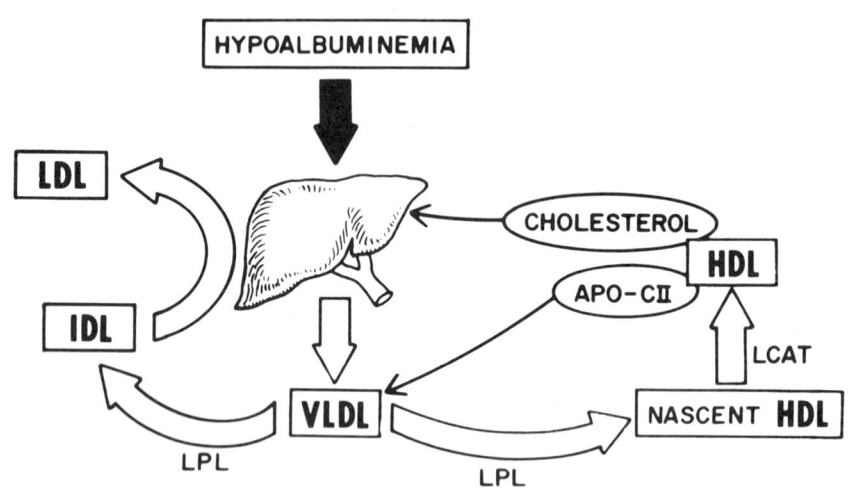

Fig 3–2.—Effects of hypoalbuminemia on lipoprotein metabolism in nephrotic syndrome. Hypoalbuminemia stimulates hepatic production of very low density lipoproteins *(VLDL)*. The concentration of other lipoproteins varies with the activity of lipoprotein lipase *(LPL)* and lecithin cholesterol acetyltransferase *(LCAT)*. (See text for details.) *LDL* = low density lipoproteins; *IDL* = intermediate density lipoproteins; *HDL* = high density lipoproteins; *APO-CII* = apoprotein CII.

liver are hydrolyzed to intermediate density lipoproteins (IDL) and nascent high density lipoproteins (HDL) by lipoprotein lipases situated in a number of extrahepatic sites including vascular endothelium, adipose tissue, and muscle. IDL are subsequently converted to low density lipoproteins (LDL) by the liver. In nephrotic patients with moderate hypoalbuminemia (2.0 to 3.0 gm/dl), VLDL produced by the liver are rapidly metabolized, so that LDL concentrations rise whereas VLDL remain relatively normal. Serum cholesterol increases but serum triglycerides remain normal. With more severe hypoalbuminemia (serum levels less than 1.0 gm/dl), VLDL accumulate and LDL concentrations fall so that serum triglyceride levels rise progressively. This changing lipoprotein profile has been attributed to the inhibition of lipoprotein lipase by free fatty acids that normally bind to albumin and accumulate in adipose tissue as the serum albumin concentration falls.[15, 16] When proteinuria is massive, urinary losses of apoprotein CII, a normal component of VLDL and a potent stimulator of lipoprotein lipase, may also contribute to the accumulation of VLDL.[16]

Apoprotein CII is transported by HDL and transferred to VLDL during the catabolic process. HDL have the additional important function of removing cholesterol from the circulation and transporting it to the liver for excretion. Since HDL have molecular sizes comparable to albumin, these important lipoproteins may be reduced in the nephrotic syndrome as a result of urinary losses. In addition, the synthesis of HDL may be decreased by accumulation of unbound lysolecithin which inhibits the synthetic enzyme lecithin-cholesterol acyltransferase (see Fig 3-2). These two mechanisms would predict a reduced concentration of HDL in patients with heavy proteinuria; however, no consistent pattern of HDL serum concentrations has been identified in the nephrotic population.

Although increased hepatic lipoprotein synthesis is the major factor accounting for hyperlipidemia in the nephrotic syndrome, there is some evidence that impaired catabolism of lipids may contribute to hyperlipidemia in this disorder. For example, studies employing infusions of labeled lipoproteins have demonstrated a reduced rate of clearance of triglycerides from the plasma of nephrotic patients.[17] As indicated above, defects in the activity of lipoprotein lipase or lecithin-cholesterol acyltransferase may play a role in the altered catabolism of lipoproteins in the nephrotic syndrome.

Lipiduria commonly accompanies hyperlipidemia in the nephrotic syndrome and gives rise to characteristic urinary sediment abnormalities (Fig 3-3). Urinary lipid droplets containing cholesterol, cho-

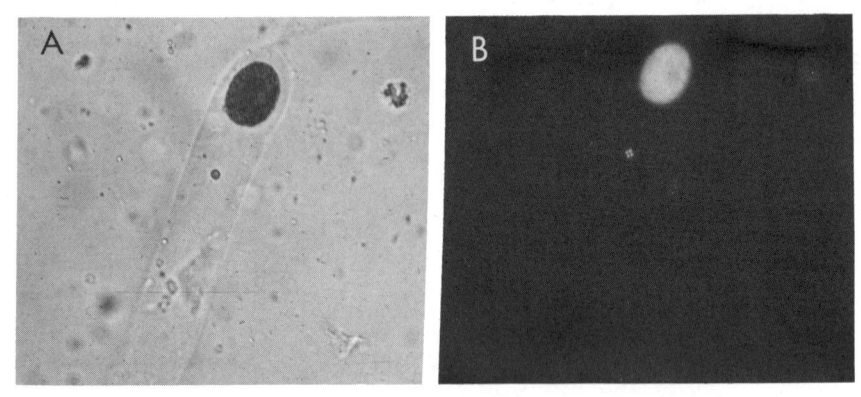

Fig 3–3.—Urine sediment from a patient with nephrotic syndrome. **A,** oval fat body and lipid droplet in a hyaline cast. **B,** same microscopic field viewed with a polarizing lens, showing birefringence of fatty material and Maltese cross appearance of the lipid droplet.

lesterol esters, or neutral fat may be present free in the urine, entrapped in casts, or enclosed within degenerating renal tubular cells ("oval fat bodies"). Cholesterol esters typically exhibit birefringence when viewed under polarized light and have a distinctive Maltese cross (or "cross patee") configuration. The exact pathways by which lipid reaches the urine in the nephrotic syndrome have not been established. Lipiduria correlates best with the magnitude of proteinuria rather than with the presence of hyperlipidemia. Since lipiduria does not occur in other forms of hyperlipoproteinemia, lipiduria in the nephrotic syndrome presumably results from increased glomerular permeability to low molecular weight, high density lipoproteins.[18] Proximal tubular cells reabsorb a fraction of the filtered lipoprotein. Following catabolism, constituent lipids may return to the tubular lumen as free fat. The proximal tubular cells may slough into the urine as oval fat bodies or retain the appearance of degenerating fat-filled cells in situ, forming the basis of the obsolete histologic designation "lipoid nephrosis."

MISCELLANEOUS CONSEQUENCES OF HEAVY PROTEINURIA

Serum Protein Abnormalities

The nephrotic syndrome is accompanied by marked alterations in the concentration of serum proteins other than albumin as illustrated in a representative serum protein electrophoresis in Figure 3–4. Hepatic synthesis of high molecular weight globulins such as fibrinogen and beta- and alpha-2-globulins is increased in nephrotic patients. The high circulating levels of these large globulins probably account for the elevated erythrocyte sedimentation rate that is frequently observed in nephrotic patients and which closely parallels the degree of proteinuria. The serum concentrations of proteins other than albumin may be reduced via urinary losses with important potential clinical consequences (Table 3–1). For example, transferrin deficiency may play a role in the development of iron deficiency anemia, a rare complication of nephrotic syndrome. Copper deficiency resulting from urinary loss of ceruloplasmin has also been described.[19] Urinary losses of immunoglobulins may result in hypogammaglobulinemia and enhanced susceptibility to infection, a phenomenon that probably contributed to the high incidence of death from bacterial sepsis in the nephrotic syndrome prior to the introduction of steroid and antibiotic therapy. Although IgG is clearly lost in the urine of nephrotic patients, urinary losses do not alone account for the pattern of hypogammaglobulinemia seen in these patients since the various subclasses of IgG appear to be decreased asymmetrically.[20] The latter

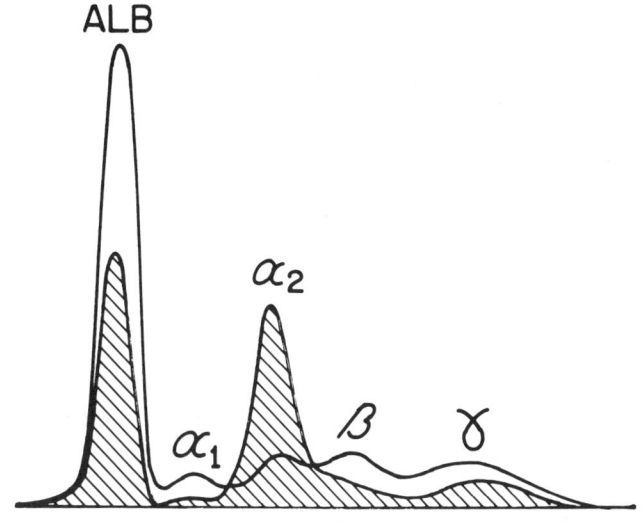

Fig 3–4.—Representative serum protein electrophoreses from a normal patient *(open curve)* and a patient with nephrotic syndrome *(hatched curve)*. (Modified from Wagoner R.D.: *The Nephrotic Syndrome: Discussions in Patient Management.* New Hyde Park, NY, Medical Examination Publishing Co., 1981, p. 10. Used by permission.)

TABLE 3–1.—SERUM PROTEIN DEFICIENCIES IN NEPHROTIC SYNDROME

PROTEIN DEFICIENCY	PHYSIOLOGIC CONSEQUENCE	CLINICAL MANIFESTATION
IgG	Hypogammaglobulinemia	Increased susceptibility to infection
Complement factor B	Defective opsonization	Increased susceptibility to infection
High density lipoprotein	Impaired cholesterol transport	Accelerated atherosclerosis
Antithrombin III	Impaired inactivation of thrombin	Thromboembolic tendency
Transferrin	Urinary loss of Fe, impaired Fe transport	Iron deficiency anemia
Ceruloplasmin	Urinary loss of Cu	Copper deficiency, ? Hemolytic tendency
Factors IX, XI, XIII	Reduced procoagulant activity	Prolonged partial thromboplastin time
Thyroxine-binding globulin	Increased T_3 resin uptake, decreased total T_4	Chemical hypothyroidism
Vitamin D-binding, globulin	Decreased 25-hydroxycholecalciferol, decreased 1,25-dihydroxycholecalciferol	Hypocalcemia, osteomalacia, secondary hyperparathyroidism

observation suggests that the nephrotic syndrome is accompanied by alterations in the synthesis or catabolism of specific IgG subclasses.

A number of hormone-binding globulins may be lost in the urine of nephrotic patients. Deficiency of thyroxine-binding globulin[21] results in a high T3 resin uptake and a low total T4 serum concentration; however, serum levels of free T4 and thyroid stimulating hormone (TSH) are usually normal and the thyroid-pituitary axis responds appropriately to free thyroxine so that most nephrotic patients remain clinically euthyroid. Loss of vitamin D-binding globulin has been implicated in a syndrome consisting of impaired gastrointestinal calcium absorption, hypocalcemia, secondary hyperparathyroidism, and osteomalacia that may complicate the nephrotic syndrome even when glomerular filtration rate is well preserved.[22, 23] Since hypocalcemia regularly accompanies hypoalbuminemia, this syndrome may be recognized in its incipient stages only by measurement of ionized calcium or by the measurement of active metabolites of vitamin D that are decreased in the presence of vitamin D-binding globulin deficiency. Factors IX, XI, and XII may be excreted in the urine of nephrotic patients. However, deficiency of these procoagulant proteins usually is outweighed by simultaneous alterations in coagulation and fibrinolytic factors that favor the development of a hypercoagulable state (see below).

Accelerated Atherosclerosis

Prolonged hyperlipidemia associated with heavy proteinuria may impose a notable risk of accelerated atherosclerosis. Studies of lipoprotein profiles in the nephrotic syndrome have demonstrated a high incidence of hyperlipoproteinemia types IIA and IIB—patterns that have generally been associated with an increased risk of cardiovascular disease.[24, 25] However, epidemiologic studies have reached conflicting conclusions regarding the incidence of cardiovascular morbidity and mortality in the nephrotic population.[26-28] Some autopsy studies suggesting a high incidence of coronary artery disease in nephrotic patients have included patients with systemic diseases such as diabetes mellitus and systemic lupus erythematosus, which may independently predispose to premature cardiovascular disease.[29] The consequences of hyperlipidemia in the nephrotic syndrome may not be similar to those in patients with idiopathic or familial hyperlipoproteinemias because serum lipid levels often rise and fall with exacerbations and remissions of proteinuria. Since some minimum critical time is presumably needed for any specific risk factor for cardiovascular disease to exert its effects, it seems unlikely that accelerated atherosclerosis would be associated with disease entities such as minimal change nephropathy, a disorder in which heavy proteinuria is often short lived. Furthermore, the lipid profile of proteinuric patients may vary depending on the severity of hypoalbuminemia, making the nephrotic syndrome a poor model for the study of the effects of any single lipid component on long-term cardiovascular morbidity. For example, a high circulating level of HDL cholesterol may protect against atherosclerosis by enhancing transport of cholesterol and preventing its accumulation in vascular endothelium. Conversely, a low HDL cholesterol level has been associated with an increased risk of cardiovascular disease. HDL concentrations in nephrotic subjects are quite variable, however, perhaps reflecting the varying severity of proteinuria and hypoalbuminemia. Although the risk of hyperlipidemia in the nephrotic syndrome remains a subject of controversy, it is clear that important variables to be considered in any future study of this phenomenon include the duration of heavy proteinuria, the nature of the underlying disease, and the constancy of specific lipoprotein profiles.

Proximal Tubular Dysfunction

A variety of abnormalities of proximal tubular function have been described in patients with nephrotic syndrome. The most common manifestations of proximal tubular dysfunction in this setting are glycosuria and aminoaciduria. However, a few patients have been described with more complete proximal tubular dysfunction manifested by Type II renal tubular acidosis and the full-blown Fanconi syndrome including glycosuria, hyperphosphaturia, aminoaciduria, hyperuricosuria, and renal potassium wasting.[30,31] Proximal tubular dysfunction appears to be much more common in children than in adults with nephrotic syndrome. The mechanisms accounting for tubular dysfunction in the nephrotic syndrome remain to be elucidated. It has been postulated that discrete tubular dysfunction reflects damage to tubular epithelial cells consequent on the reabsorption of filtered protein. Since the latter phenomenon occurs in all nephrotic patients, it seems unlikely that this is the sole explanation for proximal tubular dysfunction which occurs in the minority of patients with heavy proteinuria. Recent studies of children with idiopathic nephrotic syndrome suggest that the presence of multiple proximal tubular defects may predict a poor prognosis with a greater likelihood for the development of renal failure.[32,33]

Hyponatremia

Patients with nephrotic syndrome may exhibit impaired water excretion manifested by a tendency to develop hyponatremia. Hypoosmolality resulting from a true water excreting defect must be differentiated from spuriously low levels of serum sodium that can be seen in nephrotic patients with severe hyperlipidemia. The underlying mechanisms accounting for true water retention probably vary depending on the patient's plasma volume status. Since most studies of experimental nephrotic syndrome demonstrate a reduction in absolute proximal tubular reabsorption, impaired delivery of tubular fluid to the distal diluting segments of the nephron is not likely the explanation for the defect in urinary dilution in these patients. Rather, a reduction in absolute or "effective" plasma volume likely serves as a nonosmotic stimulus for the release of antidiuretic hormone.[34] This hypothesis is supported by water immersion studies in nephrotic subjects. Immersion in water to the neck expands plasma volume and promotes a free water diuresis in such patients.[35] Recent studies demonstrate an inverse relationship between plasma vasopressin levels and plasma volume in nephrotic subjects.[34] According to these concepts, hyponatremia may serve as an indicator of plasma volume depletion in the nephrotic syndrome. Diuretics should be used with special caution in the nephrotic subject with hyponatremia since they may exacerbate intravascular volume depletion and compound the defect in the excretion of free water.

Malnutrition

Above and beyond their constant urinary protein losses and excessive albumin catabolism, patients with persistent nephrotic syndrome may consume inadequate dietary protein due to anorexia, nausea, and vomiting. The latter gastrointestinal symptoms may reflect edema of the bowel wall. In addition, studies using ^{51}Cr-albumin have demonstrated increased gastrointestinal loss of albumin in patients with nephrotic syndrome, presumably reflecting a generalized capillary protein leak.[36] Some or all of these factors may collectively result in negative nitrogen balance. The adverse effects of such protein malnutrition are of special concern in the nephrotic child, since growth and development may be impaired. Short of inducing a remission of proteinuria, a high protein diet represents the mainstay of therapy to prevent malnutrition and growth retardation (see Chapter 6).

LIFE-THREATENING COMPLICATIONS OF HEAVY PROTEINURIA

Infection

Patients with the nephrotic syndrome have an increased susceptibility to a variety of infections. In the pre-antibiotic era, infection was the most common cause of death in patients with heavy proteinuria.[37] The bacterial organisms most frequently implicated include encapsulated species such as the pneumococcus and *Klebsiella,* as well as coliform species. Although pulmonary infections are common in all age groups, primary pneumococcal peritonitis is particularly common in children with the nephrotic syndrome. Increased susceptibility to infection has been attributed to a number of factors, including urinary losses of both IgG and complement Factor B. Deficiency of the latter factor results in defective opsonization and may account for the frequent occurrence of infections due to encapsulated bacteria. Generalized protein calorie malnutrition may impair other components of the immunologic response including cell-mediated immunity. Finally, the nephrotic patient's predisposition to infection may be compounded by the use of corticosteroids and other immunosuppressive drugs in the treatment of the underlying glomerulopathy. The development of effective antibiotics has drastically reduced the incidence of fatal infections in this patient population. Nevertheless, the patient with nephrotic syndrome should be regarded as an immunocompromised host, warranting aggressive antibiotic therapy whenever infection is suspected.

Vascular Collapse and Acute Renal Failure

Although nephrotic patients are heterogeneous in terms of their plasma volume status, massive proteinuria and profound hypoalbuminemia may reduce intravascular colloid osmotic pressure and diminish circulating plasma volume sufficiently in some patients to produce orthostatic hypotension and prerenal azotemia. In this tenuous state, any additional decline in plasma volume may precipitate frank circulatory collapse or acute renal failure. Such critical losses of intravascular volume may be induced by hemorrhage or gastrointestinal fluid losses; more often, they result from the overzealous use of diuretics in the treatment of nephrotic edema.

Acute renal failure appears to be more common in patients with minimal change nephropathy than in other forms of nephrotic syndrome, perhaps because plasma volumes are more consistently reduced in this disorder. Acute renal failure has been described in some nephrotic patients in the absence of impressive tubular changes on renal biopsy. As an alternate explanation for acute renal failure in these patients, it has been postulated that hypoalbuminemia may lead to renal interstitial edema, collapse of renal tubules, and a net decline in glomerular ultrafiltration pressure and glomerular filtration rate.[38] If this pathogenetic scheme is applicable to some patients with acute renal failure in the nephrotic syndrome, such patients would paradoxically benefit from intensification of diuretic therapy[38] or dialytic ultrafiltration.[39] Under most circumstances, diuretics should be used with special caution in nephrotic patients to avoid sudden contractions of extracellular volume.

Several other forms of renal failure warrant serious consideration when the nephrotic patient develops acute renal insufficiency. Acute renal vein thrombosis complicating nephrotic syndrome may be associated with an acute decline in renal function (see below). In addition, the nephrotic patient with hypovolemia may be predisposed to developing renal failure secondary to a variety of nephrotoxins including radiocontrast dye and drugs. Particularly noteworthy among the drugs capable of causing renal failure in the nephrotic syndrome are the nonsteroidal anti-inflammatory agents. As in other edematous disorders, the kidneys of patients with nephrotic syndrome are frequently under the influence of a variety of vasoconstrictor stimuli that are modulated by the renal production of vasodilatory prostaglandins. Inhibition of renal prostaglandin production in this setting may leave unopposed the effect of vasoconstrictor stimuli, leading to deleterious effects on renal blood flow and glomerular filtration rate. Indeed, a moderate decline in glomerular filtration rate frequently accompanies the use of nonsteroidal anti-inflammatory agents in proteinuric patients and forms the basis for their occasional use in reducing proteinuria in patients with persistent nephrotic syndrome[40] (see Chapter 6). Unfortunately, severe and sometimes irreversible renal failure may complicate the use of these agents,[41-43] suggesting that such drugs should be used with extreme caution in nephrotic patients. Renal failure resulting from a functional decline in renal blood flow induced by nonsteroidal anti-inflammatory drugs must be differentiated from the rare, presumably idiosyncratic form of acute renal failure that occasionally complicates their use. In this latter entity, nonsteroidal agents appear to be the cause of the nephrotic syndrome and concomitant acute renal failure. This unique renal syndrome is manifest pathologically by interstitial nephritis and foot process fusion with minimal or no glomerular changes on light microscopy[44, 45] (see Chapter 4). Finally, acute renal failure due to allergic interstitial nephritis is an uncommon but potentially serious complication of diuretic therapy in the nephrotic syndrome.[46] This complication should be considered if renal function deteriorates while the patient is receiving diuretics—especially if rash, eosinophilia, or eosinophiluria are present.

Thromboembolism

An association between the nephrotic syndrome and renal vein thrombosis as well as other thromboembolic phenomena has been appreciated since the nineteenth century. For many decades renal vein thrombosis was considered an infrequent *cause* of nephrotic syndrome. This belief was perpetuated by the occasional occurrence of heavy proteinuria in patients with severe cardiac failure or constrictive pericarditis, conditions characterized by renal venous hypertension. Renal vein thrombosis currently is regarded as a complication rather than a cause of the nephrotic syndrome. Evidence favoring this view can be summarized as follows: First, experimental elevation of renal venous pressure by occlusion of the renal vein does not produce heavy proteinuria unless contralateral nephrectomy is performed. Second, renal vein thrombosis occurs in animal models of nephrotic syndrome with an incidence as high as 20%. Third, patients with renal vein occlusion secondary to tumors or extension of clot from the vena cava do not have proteinuria. Fourth, nephrotic patients with unilateral renal vein thrombosis have bilateral proteinuria.[47]

Although the apparent predilection for thrombosis of the renal veins remains largely unexplained, it is now generally believed that the high incidence of renal vein thrombosis in patients with the nephrotic syndrome reflects a generalized tendency to develop thromboembolism resulting from a hypercoagulable state. Indeed, the incidence of thromboembolic events such as peripheral venous thrombophlebitis and pulmonary emboli is increased in nephrotic patients in the absence of renal vein thrombi. The pathogenesis of hypercoagulability in the nephrotic syndrome probably is multifactorial (Fig 3–5). Levels of fibrinogen, factors V, VII, VIII, and X are frequently elevated.[48, 49] However, it is unlikely that increased levels of coagulation factors alone cause hypercoagulability, since these factors are normally present in great excess, only a small proportion being activated during thrombus formation. Increased urinary excretion of antithrombin III, a potent thrombolytic protein with a molecular weight similar to albumin, may play a role in the thrombotic tendency of some patients.[50, 51] If large quantities of antithrombin III are lost in the urine, renal venous concentrations of this substance would be lower than in any other part of the circulation, a phenomenon that

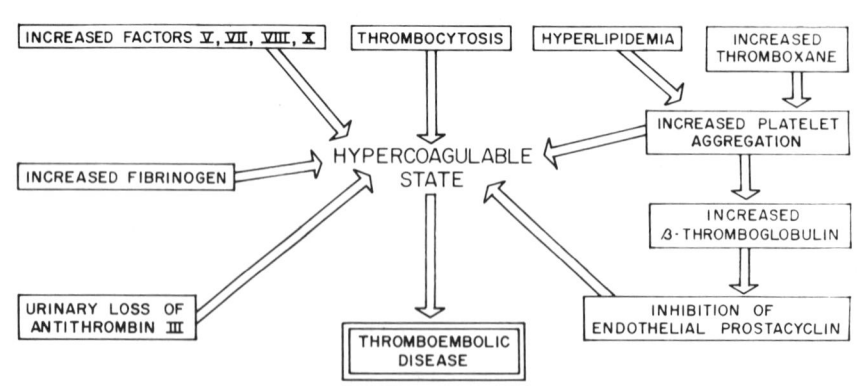

Fig 3–5.—Mechanisms of hypercoagulability and thromboembolism in the nephrotic syndrome.

might explain the tendency for thrombus to form in the renal veins. Thrombocytosis has occasionally been described in the nephrotic syndrome. Recent evidence suggests that the platelets of nephrotic patients are hyperaggregable,[52–54] perhaps as the result of hyperlipoproteinemia which may alter the lipid composition of the platelet membrane. Platelet hyperaggregability in the nephrotic syndrome is inversely related to the serum albumin concentration. Albumin binds arachidonic acid and limits its conversion to thromboxane A_2, a potent stimulator of platelet aggregation.[55, 56] Thus, a normal albumin concentration may provide an important modulating influence on platelet aggregation. Conversely, enhanced production of thromboxane A_2 in hypoalbuminemic patients may contribute to platelet hyperaggregability,[55, 57] a hypothesis supported by the reversal of platelet aggregation following the infusion of albumin.[52] Aggregating platelets release beta-thromboglobulin, which may further contribute to hypercoagulability by inhibiting the synthesis of prostacyclin in the vascular endothelium.[58]

Considering renal vein thrombosis alone, the incidence of thromboembolism varies from 2% to 29% in recent series of patients with the nephrotic syndrome.[59–61] Renal vein thrombosis is thought to be particularly common in patients with membranous glomerulopathy, but this observation may simply reflect the fact that membranous glomerulopathy is the most common underlying glomerular lesion in adults with idiopathic nephrotic syndrome. Indeed, a variety of glomerular lesions has been associated with renal vein thrombosis (Table 3–2). Diabetic nephropathy is a conspicuously rare cause of renal vein thrombosis in most large series, an observation that remains unexplained since diabetic glomerulosclerosis represents the most common form of secondary nephrotic syndrome.

The large variation in the reported frequency of renal vein thrombosis may reflect the aggressiveness with which the diagnosis of this complication is pursued. Renal vein thrombosis is easily recognized when the nephrotic patient presents with acute flank pain, hematuria and a sudden deterioration of renal function. In such cases, intravenous pyelography characteristically reveals unilateral renal enlargement, pelvocalyceal irregularities, or ureteral notching from enlarged venous collaterals. Chronic asymptomatic renal vein thrombosis is the more common mode of clinical presentation, however, especially in adults.[59] In such patients, the intravenous pyelogram frequently is normal and the condition may go unnoticed until the patient develops progressive deterioration of renal function or pulmonary emboli. Until discrepancies in the reported frequency of thromboembolic complica-

TABLE 3–2.—ETIOLOGY OF THE NEPHROTIC SYNDROME: INCIDENCE OF RENAL VEIN THROMBOSIS IN 151 CASES*

RENAL DIAGNOSIS	NO. OF PATIENTS WITH RENAL VEIN THROMBOSIS	NO. OF PATIENTS WITHOUT RENAL VEIN THROMBOSIS	TOTAL
Membranous nephropathy	20	49	69
Membranoproliferative glomerulonephritis	6	21	27
Lipoid nephrosis	2	8	10
Rapidly progressive glomerulonephritis	1	1	2
Amyloidosis	1	5	6
Focal sclerosis	1	3	4
Renal sarcoidosis	1	0	1
Lupus nephritis	1	10	11
Diabetic nephropathy	0	15	15
Focal glomerulonephritis	0	3	3
Acute poststreptococcal glomerulonephritis	0	2	2
End-stage renal disease	0	1	1
TOTALS	33	118	151

*From Llach.[59]

tions are clarified by further data, the routine use of venography, intravenous pyelography, or empiric anticoagulant therapy in all patients with nephrotic syndrome does not seem warranted (see Chapter 6).

Treatment of renal vein thrombosis consists of systemic anticoagulation. Anticoagulant therapy is effective in preventing new thromboembolic events but apparently has little effect on the restoration of compromised renal function in those patients with renal vein thrombosis complicated by renal insufficiency. The appropriate duration of anticoagulation therapy remains open to question. In patients with persistent nephrotic syndrome, it may be reasonable to continue anticoagulant therapy so long as heavy proteinuria persists. A three- to six-month course of oral anticoagulant therapy with warfarin is probably adequate for the treatment of isolated renal vein thrombosis in patients who sustain a remission from heavy proteinuria. Since increased platelet aggregability appears to be a major factor in the hypercoagulable state associated with nephrotic syndrome, antiplatelet agents may be reasonable alternatives for long-term therapy; however, the efficacy of such agents in preventing recurrent thromboembolic episodes has not been adequately tested. Fibrinolytic agents such as streptokinase have been used successfully in the treatment of acute renal vein thrombosis,[62, 63] but the safety and efficacy of this form of thrombolytic therapy have not been formally compared to conventional anticoagulant therapy.

REFERENCES

1. Jensen H., Rossing N., Anderson S.B., et al.: Albumin metabolism in the nephrotic syndrome in adults. *Clin. Sci.* 33:445, 1967.
2. Blahd W.H., Fields M., Goldman R.: The turnover rate of serum albumin in the nephrotic syndrome as determined by I^{131}-labelled albumin. *J. Lab. Clin. Med.* 46:747, 1955.
3. Kaitz A.L.: Albumin metabolism in nephrotic adults. *J. Lab. Clin. Med.* 53:186, 1959.
4. Katz J., Bonorris G., Sellers A.L.: Albumin metabolism in aminonucleoside nephrotic rats. *J. Lab. Clin. Med.* 62:910, 1963.
5. Katz J., Sellers A.L., Bonorris G.: Effect of nephrectomy on plasma albumin catabolism in experimental nephrosis. *J. Lab. Clin. Med.* 63:680, 1964.
6. Hardwicke J., Squire J.R.: The relationship between plasma albumin concentration and protein excretion in patients with proteinuria. *Clin. Sci.* 14:509, 1955.
7. Ruszynak J., Foldi M., Szabo G.: Lymphocytes and Lymph Circulation, ed. 2. Oxford, Pergamon Press, 1967.
8. Benhold H., Klaus D., Scheurlen P.G.: Volume regulation and renal function in analbuminemia. *Lancet* 2:1169, 1960.
9. Dorhout Mees E.J., Roos J.C., Boer P., et al.: Observations on edema formation in the nephrotic syndrome in adults with minimal lesions. *Am. J. Med.* 67:378, 1979.
10. Miltzer J.K., Keim H.J., Laragh J.H., et al.: Nephrotic syndrome: Vasoconstriction and hypervolemic types indicated by renin-sodium profiling. *Ann. Intern. Med.* 91:688, 1979.
11. Bernard D.B., Alexander E.A., Couser W.G., et al.: Renal sodium retention during volume expansion in experimental nephrotic syndrome. *Kidney Int.* 14:478, 1978.
12. Marsh J.B., Sparks C.E.: Hepatic secretion of lipoproteins in the rat and the effects of experimental nephrosis. *J. Clin. Invest.* 64:1229, 1979.
13. Baxter J.H., Goodman H.C., Allen J.C.: Effects of infusions of serum albumin on serum lipids and lipoproteins in nephrosis. *J. Clin. Invest.* 40:490, 1961.
14. Allen J.C., Baxter J.H., Goodman H.C.: Effects of dextran, polyvinylpyrrolidone and gammaglobulin on the hyperlipidemia of experimental nephrosis. *J. Clin. Invest.* 40:499, 1961.
15. Baxter J.H.: Hyperlipoproteinemia in nephrosis. *Arch. Intern. Med.* 109:146, 1962.
16. Kashyap M.L., Srivastava L.S., Hynd B.A., et al.: Apolipoprotein CII and lipoprotein lipase in human nephrotic syndrome. *Atherosclerosis* 35:29, 1980.
17. McKenzie I.F.C., Nestle P.J.: Studies on the turnover of triglyceride and esterified cholesterol in subjects with the nephrotic syndrome. *J. Clin. Invest.* 47:685, 1968.
18. Zimmer J.G., Dewey R., Waterhouse C., et al.: The origin and nature of anisotropic urinary lipids in the nephrotic syndrome. *Ann. Intern. Med.* 54:205, 1961.
19. Cartwright G.E., Gubler C.J., Wintrobe M.M.: Studies on copper metabolism: XI. Copper and iron metabolism in the nephrotic syndrome. *J. Clin. Invest.* 33:685, 1954.
20. Shakib F., Hardwicke J., Stanworth D.R., et al.: Asymmetric depression in the serum of IgG subclasses in patients with nephrotic syndrome. *Clin. Exp. Immunol.* 28:506, 1977.
21. Musa B.U., Seal U.S., Doe R.P.: Excretion of corticosteroid-binding globulin and total protein in adult males with nephrosis: effect of sex hormones. *J. Clin. Endocrinol. Metab.* 27:768, 1967.
22. Malluche H.H., Goldstein D.A., Massry S.G.: Osteomalacia and hyperparathyroid bone disease in patients with nephrotic syndrome. *J. Clin. Invest.* 63:494, 1979.

23. Schmidt-Gayk H., Schmitt W., Grawunder C., et al.: 25-hydroxy-vitamin D in nephrotic syndrome. *Lancet* 2:105, 1977.
24. Chopra J.S., Mallick N.P., Stone M.C.: Hyperlipoproteinemias in nephrotic syndrome. *Lancet* 1:317, 1971.
25. Newmark S.R., Anderson C.F., Donadio J.V., et al.: Lipoprotein profiles in adult nephrotics. *Mayo Clin. Proc.* 50:359, 1975.
26. Mallick N.P., Short C.D.: The nephrotic syndrome and ischaemic heart disease. *Nephron* 27:54, 1981.
27. Wass U., Cameron J.S.: Cardiovascular disease and the nephrotic syndrome: The other side of the coin. *Nephron* 27:58, 1981.
28. Wass V.J., Jarrett R.J., Chilvers C., et al.: Does the nephrotic syndrome increase the risk of cardiovascular disease? *Lancet* 2:664, 1979.
29. Curry R.G., Roberts W.C.: Status of the coronary arteries in the nephrotic syndrome. *Am. J. Med.* 63:183, 1977.
30. Stickler G.B., Hayles A.B., Power M.H., et al.: Renal tubular dysfunction complicating the nephrotic syndrome. *Pediatrics* 26:75, 1969.
31. Stanbury S.W., Macauley D.: Defects of renal tubular function in the nephrotic syndrome. *Q. J. Med.* 26:7, 1957.
32. Bouissou F., Barthe P.L., Pierragi M.: Severe idiopathic nephrotic syndrome with tubular dysfunction (report of nine pediatric cases). *Clin. Nephrol.* 14:135, 1980.
33. McVicar M., Exeni R., Susin M.: Nephrotic syndrome and multiple tubular defects in children: an early sign of focal segmental glomerulosclerosis. *J. Pediatr.* 97:918, 1980.
34. Usberti M., Federico S., Meccariello S., et al.: Role of plasma vasopressin in the impairment of water excretion in nephrotic syndrome. *Kidney Int.* 25:422, 1984.
35. Berlyne G.M., Brown C., Adler A.: Water immersion in the nephrotic syndrome. *Arch. Intern. Med.* 141:1275, 1981.
36. Schultze G., Ahuja S., Faber U., et al.: Gastrointestinal protein loss in the nephrotic syndrome studied with ^{51}Cr-albumin. *Nephron* 25:277, 1980.
37. Arneil G.C.: 164 children with nephrosis. *Lancet* 2:1103, 1961.
38. Lowenstein J., Schacht R.G., Baldwin D.J.: Renal failure in minimal change nephrotic syndrome. *Am. J. Med.* 70:227, 1981.
39. Sjoberg R.J., McMillan U.M., Bartram L.S., et al.: Renal failure with minimal change nephrotic syndrome: reversal with hemodialysis. *Clin. Nephrol.* 20:98, 1983.
40. Arisz L., Donker A.J.M., Brentjens R.J.H., et al.: The effect of indomethacin on proteinuria and kidney function in the nephrotic syndrome. *Acta Med. Scand.* 199:121, 1976.
41. Walshe J.J., Venuto R.C.: Acute oliguric renal failure induced by indomethacin: possible mechamism. *Ann. Intern. Med.* 91:47, 1979.
42. Gary N.E., Dodelson R., Eisinger R.P.: Indomethacin-associated acute renal failure. *Am. J. Med.* 69:135, 1980.
43. McCarthy J.T., Torres V.E., Romero J.C., et al.: Acute intrinsic renal failure induced by indomethacin: role of prostaglandin synthetase inhibition. *Mayo Clin. Proc.* 57:289, 1982.
44. Brezin J.H., Katz S.M., Schwartz A.B., et al.: Reversible renal failure and nephrotic syndrome associated with nonsteroidal anti-inflammatory drugs. *N. Engl. J. Med.* 301:1271, 1979.
45. Finkelstein A., Fraley D.S., Feldman H.A., et al.: Fenoprofen nephropathy: Lipoid nephrosis and interstitial nephritis. *Am. J. Med.* 72:81, 1982.
46. Lyons H., Pinn V.W., Cortell S., et al.: Allergic interstitial nephritis causing reversible renal failure in four patients with idiopathic nephrotic syndrome. *N. Engl. J. Med.* 288:124, 1973.
47. Kassirer J.P.: Thrombosis and embolism of the renal vessels, in Early L.E., Gottschalk C.W. (eds.): *Strauss and Welt's Diseases of the Kidney*. Boston, Little, Brown & Co., 1979.

48. Thompson C., Forbes C.D., Prentice C.E.M., et al.: Changes in blood coagulation and fibrinolysis in the nephrotic syndrome. *Q. J. Med.* 43:399, 1974.
49. Kendall A.G., Lohman R.C., Dossetor J.B.: Nephrotic syndrome. A hypercoagulable state. *Arch. Intern. Med.* 127:1021, 1971.
50. Kauffman R., Veltkamp J., Tilberg N., et al.: Acquired antithrombin III deficiency and thrombosis in the nephrotic syndrome. *Am. J. Med.* 65:607, 1978
51. Vaziri N.D., Paule P., Tochey J., et al.: Acquired deficiency and urinary excretion of antithrombin III in nephrotic syndrome. *Arch. Intern. Med.* 144:1802, 1984.
52. Remuzzi G., Mecca G., Marchesi D., et al.: Platelet hyperaggregability and the nephrotic syndrome. *Thromb. Res.* 16:345, 1979.
53. Tomura S., Ida T., Kuriyama R., et al.: Activation of platelets in patients with chronic proliferative glomerulonephritis and the nephrotic syndrome. *Br. J. Haematol.* 52:69, 1982.
54. Kuhlmann U., Steurer J., Rhyner K., et al.: Platelet aggregation and -thromboglobulin levels in nephrotic patients with and without thrombosis. *Clin. Nephrol.* 15:229, 1981.
55. Schieppati A., Dodesini P., Benigni A., et al.: The metabolism of arachidonic induced human platelet aggregation and prostaglandin formation. *Prostaglandins* 4:863, 1973.
56. Bills T.K., Smith J.B., Silver M.J.: Platelet uptake, release, and oxidation of ^{14}C arachidonic acid, in Smith J.B., Kocsis J.J. (eds.): *Prostaglandins in Hematology.* New York, Spectrum Publications, 1977, pp. 27–55.
57. Schieppati A., Dodesini P., Benigni A., et al.: The metabolism of arachidonic acid by platelets in nephrotic syndrome. *Kidney Int.* 25:671, 1984.
58. Adler A.J., Lundin A.P., Feinroth M.V., et al.: Beta-thromboglobulin levels in nephrotic syndrome. *Am. J. Med.* 69:551, 1980.
59. Llach F., Papper S., Massry S.G.: The clinical spectrum of renal vein thrombosis: acute and chronic. *Am. J. Med.* 69:819, 1981.
60. Andrassy K., Ritz E., Bommer J.: Hypercoagulability in the nephrotic syndrome. *Klin. Wochenschr.* 58:1029, 1980.
61. Pohl M.A., MacLaurin J.P., Alfidi R.J.: Renal vein thrombosis and the nephrotic syndrome. *Abstracts Am. Soc. Neph.* 10:20A, 1977.
62. Crowley J.P., Matarese R.A., Quevedo S.F., et al.: Fibrinolytic therapy for bilateral renal vein thrombosis. *Arch. Intern. Med.* 144:159, 1984.
63. Burrow C.R., Walker W.G., Bell W.R., et al.: Streptokinase salvage of renal function after renal vein thrombosis. *Ann. Intern. Med.* 100:237, 1984.

4 Disorders Associated With Secondary Nephrotic Syndrome

THE NEPHROTIC SYNDROME can occur as a consequence of a primary glomerulopathy or as a manifestation of one of a variety of systemic disorders. Because differentiation of primary and secondary forms of nephrotic syndrome has important diagnostic and therapeutic implications, the physician must consider the various causes of the secondary nephrotic syndrome in any patient with heavy proteinuria. The disorders shown in Table 4–1 have all been linked to the development of the nephrotic syndrome. A careful history, physical examination, urinalysis, and selected laboratory studies allow the physician to classify the vast majority of patients with the nephrotic syndrome into secondary or primary forms (see Chapter 6). In this chapter we discuss the epidemiology, pathological characteristics, pathophysiology, clinical features, and management issues of the disorders most frequently associated with the secondary nephrotic syndrome.

DIABETES MELLITUS

Epidemiology

Diabetic nephropathy, characterized by proteinuria and inexorable progression to end stage renal disease (ESRD), occurs in 40% to 50% of type I diabetics and in approximately 10% to 20% of type II diabetics.[1-5] Because the prevalence of type II diabetes is far greater than that of type I diabetes, the absolute number of patients developing ESRD from each population is about equal.[6] Diabetic glomerulosclerosis is the most common cause of the secondary nephrotic syndrome. In most centers, diabetic nephropathy accounts for approximately

TABLE 4–1.—Causes of the Secondary Nephrotic Syndrome

Multisystem Disorders	Drugs
Diabetes mellitus	Gold salts
Systemic lupus erythematosus	Penicillamine
Amyloidosis	Nonsteroidal anti-inflammatory drugs
Wegener's granulomatosis	
Sickle cell anemia	Captopril
Cryoglobulinemia	"Street" heroin
Henoch-Schönlein purpura	Lithium
Polyarteritis nodosa	Chlorpropamide
Neoplastic Disorders	Trimethadione
Hodgkin's disease	*Miscellaneous*
Carcinoma	Alport's Syndrome
Lymphoma	Preeclampsia
Leukemia	Chronic Allograft Rejection
Light chain nephropathy	Vesicoureteral Reflux
Infectious Diseases	Renal Artery Stenosis
Poststreptococcal glomerulonephritis	
Bacterial endocarditis	
Hepatitis B	
Secondary syphilis	
Malaria	
Schistosomiasis	

30% of all patients with ESRD. Of patients ultimately requiring dialysis because of diabetic renal disease, as many as 70% to 75% will manifest nephrotic range proteinuria at some time during their clinical course.[2]

Pathology

Although the clinical course of patients with type I and type II diabetes may differ, renal pathologic changes are identical. Examination of renal tissue from patients with diabetic nephropathy reveals a spectrum of histologic changes including vascular, interstitial, and glomerular lesions. The combined presence of afferent and efferent arteriolar hyalinosis is characteristic of diabetic renal disease.[3] This lesion, characterized by infiltration of vessel walls with PAS positive material, is the earliest documented histologic change in normal kidneys transplanted into diabetic recipients.[7] Chronic interstitial nephritis, interstitial and periglomerular fibrosis, and papillary necrosis are common but nonspecific features of diabetic nephropathy.

Neither interstitial nor vascular lesions account for the frequent occurrence of the nephrotic syndrome in diabetic nephropathy. Glomerular involvement is the hallmark of diabetic renal disease and is responsible for the heavy proteinuria. The earliest glomerular changes consist of an increase in mesangial matrix and thickening of the glomerular basement membrane (GBM).[5, 8] The latter finding is similar to the widening of capillary basement membranes found in other vascular beds. These early glomerular abnormalities antedate the onset of clinically apparent nephropathy by several years. As diabetic nephropathy progresses, the mesangial and basement membrane changes evolve into the characteristic histologic changes of diabetic glomerulosclerosis. Diabetic glomerulosclerosis, characterized histologically by marked thickening of the GBM and expansion of the mesangial matrix (Fig 4–1), is generally associated with overt proteinuria. In about 20% of patients with diabetic glomerulosclerosis, mesangial expansion progresses to nodule formation resulting in nodular intercapillary glomerulosclerosis (Fig 4–2). Nodular glomerulosclerosis or *Kimmelstiel Wilson disease* has been considered pathognomonic of diabetic nephropathy; however, a similar light microscopic picture has been described in amyloidosis, membranoproliferative glomerulonephritis, and light chain nephropathy.[9] Distinguishing these latter entities from diabetic nephropathy often requires immunofluorescent and electron microscopic examination of biopsy specimens.

Immunofluorescent examination of renal tissue from patients with diabetic nephropathy usually reveals no staining for immunoglobulins or complement. Occasionally, a fine linear deposition of IgG is observed within the GBM. In all likelihood, this represents nonspecific trapping of IgG since albumin is found in a similar distribution

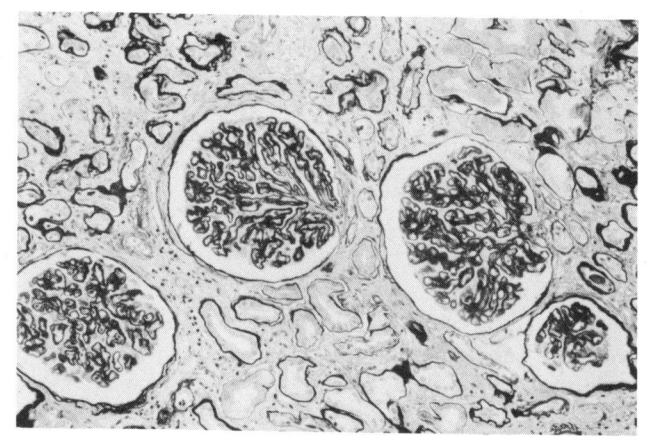

Fig 4–1.—Periodic acid-Schiff-stained renal biopsy specimen demonstrating diffuse diabetic glomerulosclerosis. There is moderate thickening of the GBM and expansion of the mesangial matrix.

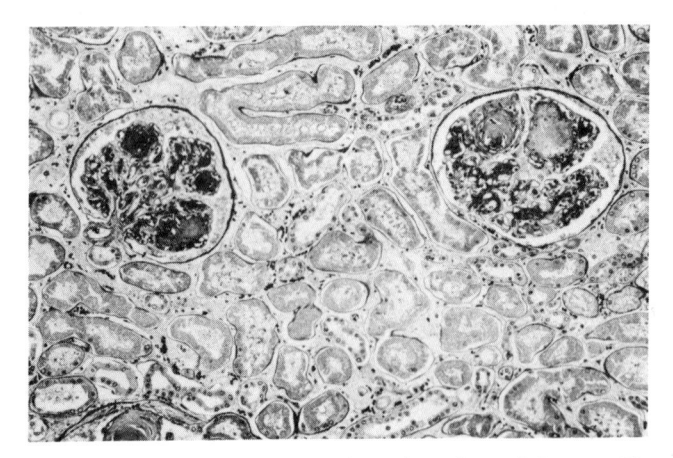

Fig 4–2.—Periodic acid-Schiff-stained section of renal tissue with nodular intercapillary glomerulosclerosis or Kimmelsteil Wilson disease. A progressive increase in mesangial matrix has resulted in the formation of characteristic mesangial nodules.

and circulating anti-GBM antibody cannot be demonstrated. Electron microscopy in diabetic glomerulosclerosis shows thickening of the GBM, expansion of the mesangial matrix with nodule formation in some cases, and effacement or "fusion" of the epithelial foot processes in patients with heavy proteinuria.[5]

Extensive efforts to identify a specific biochemical abnormality responsible for the development of diabetic glomerulosclerosis have provided conflicting data. Early studies suggested that diabetic GBM contained increased amounts of hydroxylysine, glucose, and galactose and a reduced content of lysine. But more recent investigations have failed to verify these initial results.[10] Currently the biochemical abnormality responsible for the development of diabetic glomerulosclerosis is unknown.

Pathophysiology

The precise pathophysiologic mechanisms underlying the development of diabetic nephropathy are incompletely understood. Experimental work has clearly shown that diabetic renal disease is the product of an abnormal internal milieu resulting from insulin lack, hyperglycemia, or both. In animals with experimentally induced diabetes, diabetic nephropathy can be prevented by pancreatic islet cell transplantation. Moreover, histologically established diabetic nephropathy can be reversed by transplantation of diabetic kidneys into normal recipients.[5] Whether the histologic and functional abnormalities result from insulin lack with consequent derangement of mesangial matrix and GBM synthesis or from the direct toxicity of glycosylated proteins requires further clarification.[11] It is puzzling that only one third to one half of type I diabetics develop diabetic nephropathy at all. Despite large gaps in our knowledge of the pathophysiology of diabetic nephropathy, recent studies have documented sequential changes in renal function during the course of the disease, examined the mechanisms of proteinuria, and stressed the importance of intraglomerular hemodynamic alterations as contributing factors in the decline of glomerular filtration rate (GFR). Most of these studies have been conducted in type I diabetes but, with few exceptions, are applicable to type II diabetes as well.

Newly diagnosed type I diabetics have supernormal GFRs.[5, 8, 12, 13] Insulin administration reduces blood glucose and GFR toward normal, but GFR remains mildly increased compared to normal subjects until the onset of fixed proteinuria; thereafter, it declines at an approximate rate of 1 ml/minute/month.[8] Kidney size is also increased at the outset in type I diabetes and is the morphologic correlate of the increase in GFR. The etiology of glomerular hyperfunction in early type I diabetes is unknown. It does not appear to be the result of hyperglycemia per se, since the supernormal GFR found in type I diabetes does not occur in type II diabetes.[5, 8, 12] Glomerular hyperfiltration was once regarded as an interesting physiologic epiphenomenon in diabetes, but recent work suggests that it may play an important role in the ultimate decline in renal function (see below).[13]

Proteinuria is an essential element of diabetic nephropathy. Even before clinically detectable proteinuria occurs, increments in urinary albumin excretion are demonstrable by sensitive radioimmunoassay techniques. Mogensen[8] and Viberti and co-workers[14, 15] have shown that this microalbuminuria precedes fixed proteinuria and can be normalized by strict glycemic control. The sharp decrease in microalbuminuria during one to three days of continuous subcutaneous insulin administration suggests a functional rather than structural basis for the defect.[14] Microalbuminuria accurately predicts the ultimate development of clinical proteinuria and the eventual relentless decline in GFR.[16]

Studies by Myers and associates[17, 18] have identified possible mechanisms responsible for proteinuria in diabetic nephropathy. These workers have compared renal excretion of infused dextran, albumin, and IgG in diabetic subjects and normal controls and found a restriction of dextran filtration associated with enhanced excretion of albumin in early diabetic nephropathy. By contrast, patients with established proteinuria exhibited an increased fractional clearance of dextran in addition to the excretion of albumin and larger molecular weight proteins (see Chapter 2). These data support the concept that microalbuminuria in early diabetic nephropathy is the result of a charge-selective defect in the diabetic GBM, a possible consequence of its reduced sialic acid and heparan sulfate content.[13] On the other hand, focal disruption or distortion of the GBM in established nephropathy may result in size-selective defects, filtration of large molecular weight substances and heavy proteinuria. Taken together, these studies suggest that any attempt to prevent development of diabetic nephropathy should focus on the identification and intensive treatment of patients with microalbuminuria. Strict glycemic control is probably less beneficial in reversing the glomerular structural abnormalities of patients with established heavy proteinuria.

Insulin lack and hyperglycemia are not the sole determinants of the development and progression of diabetic nephropathy; altered intraglomerular hemodynamics probably play a contributing role. There is now substantial clinical and experimental evidence suggesting that increased glomerular perfusion pressure causes progressive glomerular sclerosis, accelerating the loss of renal function in renal insufficiency of any cause.[19] In this regard, Hostetter and his co-workers have provided compelling evidence that the supernormal GFR in early diabetes plays an important role in the progression, if not the initiation, of diabetic nephropathy.[13] It seems likely that hemody-

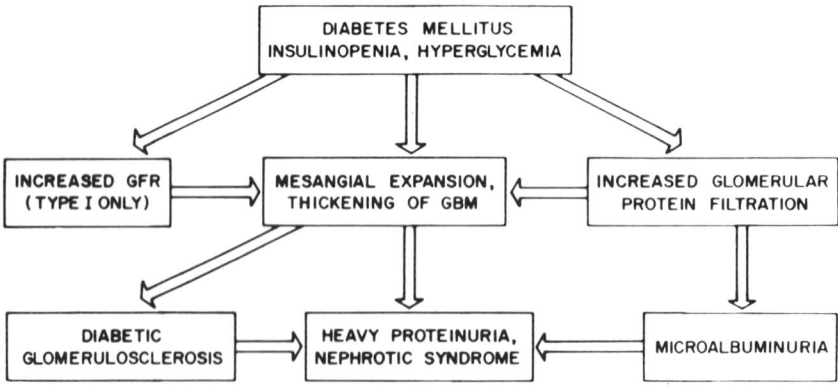

Fig 4-3.—Postulated mechanisms in the pathogenesis of diabetic nephropathy.

namic alterations are modulating influences, rather than fundamental determinants of the development of diabetic nephropathy.[20]

Figure 4–3 summarizes a hypothetical sequence of events in the development of diabetic nephropathy. According to this scheme, some hormonal or metabolic defect associated with the diabetic state (e.g., insulinopenia, hyperglycemia, etc.) results in progressive thickening of the GBM, expansion of the mesangial matrix, and increased protein filtration. The initial increase in protein filtration, manifest as microalbuminuria, is selective and potentially reversible with tight control of blood glucose. Worsening metabolic control results in increasing filtration of protein and deposition of circulating proteins within the mesangium. In type I diabetes, the increase in glomerular capillary pressure resulting from a supernormal GFR is a further stimulus to mesangial expansion and thickening of the GBM. The eventual development of glomerulosclerosis produces nonselective heavy proteinuria and further mesangial protein deposition.

Clinical Features

Although the histological manifestations are identical in patients with type I and type II diabetes, the clinical course of diabetic nephropathy differs in these two subgroups. Patients with type II diabetes have an earlier onset of proteinuria, a lesser prevalence of nephrotic syndrome and slower progression to renal insufficiency compared to their type I counterparts.[3] Furthermore, only 10% to 20% of maturity onset diabetics develop ESRD, compared to 40% to 50% of those with juvenile onset diabetes. Our knowledge regarding the natural history of diabetic nephropathy is drawn primarily from studies of patients with type I diabetes because of the ease in determining the onset of this disorder. However, with few noted exceptions, the following discussion is applicable to both type I and type II diabetes.

Microalbuminuria is the earliest sign of renal involvement in diabetes mellitus. Mogensen and his colleagues followed 43 diabetic subjects for 7 to 14 years.[21] Of 14 patients with microalbuminuria at the onset, 12 developed clinically detectable proteinuria (>500 mg/24 hours), whereas none of the 29 without microalbuminuria progressed to fixed proteinuria. Proteinuria exceeding 300 to 500 mg/24 hours occurs on average after 16 to 17 years of type I diabetes[2, 5, 22] and after 10 to 12 years of type II diabetes.[2] Proteinuria increases over the ensuing years so that 45% to 80% of type I diabetics with diabetic

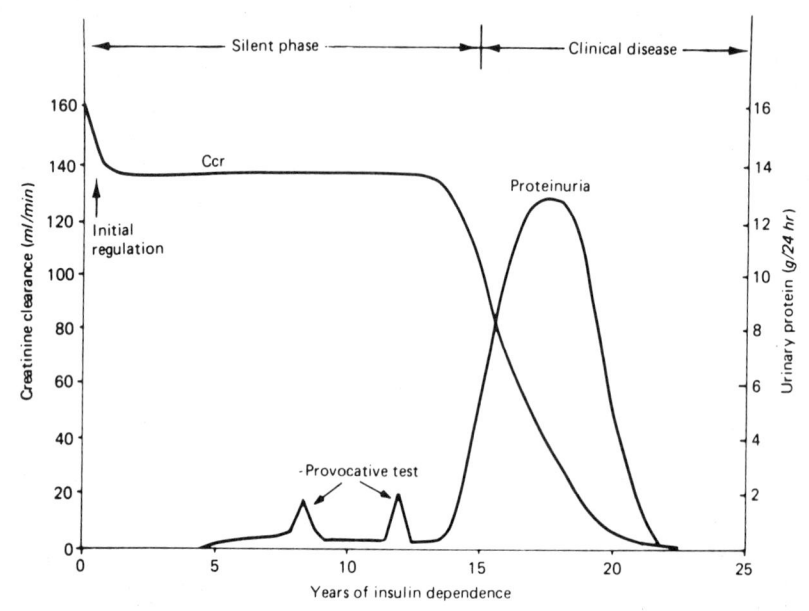

Fig 4–4.—Clinical course of type I diabetic nephropathy. Supernormal creatinine clearance *(Ccr)* is usual before the development of overt proteinuria. Proteinuria typically precedes azotemia. Interval between onset of insulin dependence and end-stage renal failure is typically 20 years. (Courtesy of Friedman E.A.: *Kidney Int.* 21:780, 1982.)

nephropathy and 5% to 70% of type II diabetics ultimately develop nephrotic range proteinuria.[2, 3] The discrepant estimates regarding the prevalence of the nephrotic syndrome in maturity onset diabetes are difficult to reconcile but may be due to selection criteria, length of observation, or other undefined factors.

Fixed and increasing proteinuria is an ominous sign and a harbinger of ultimate progression to ESRD. Once clinically overt proteinuria develops in patients with insulin dependent diabetes, GFR declines at a constant rate of approximately 1/ml/minute/month (range 0.6 to 2.5 ml/minute/month).[5, 23] Early renal insufficiency occurs approximately 2 years after the development of overt proteinuria and ESRD within 5 to 6 years.[22] Thus, the clinical course of at least type I diabetic nephropathy is characterized by a long latent period with a supernormal GFR, followed by the relatively rapid development of proteinuria, nephrotic syndrome, azotemia, and ESRD (Fig 4–4). A qualitatively similar but quantitatively different course may be seen in maturity onset diabetic nephropathy.[2, 3]

Retinopathy, neuropathy, hypertension, and vascular disease are frequent concomitants of clinically overt diabetic nephropathy. Over 60% of patients will have diabetic retinopathy when renal disease is first diagnosed; in the majority of the remainder, retinal involvement develops with progression to ESRD.[2, 5, 11, 24] Thus, although retinopathy is generally observed with the clinical onset of diabetic nephropathy, it is not an invariable accompaniment and its absence should not exclude the diagnosis. Hypertension occurs in over 50% of patients with diabetic nephropathy and correlates with the decrement in GFR.[3, 25] Hypertension rarely antedates clinically overt nephropathy, suggesting that the increase in blood pressure is largely the result of renal sodium retention. Hypertension, reduced sodium excretion, and diabetic microvascular disease together account for the frequent episodes of congestive heart failure that characterize the clinical course of the diabetic with declining renal function.

Examination of the urine sediment in patients with diabetic nephropathy reveals a spectrum of abnormalities. Many patients have essentially normal findings. However, asymptomatic bacteruria (45%), hematuria and leukocyturia (20% to 30%), and even RBC casts (10%) are found in a minority of patients.[2, 3, 26] Diabetics with the full-blown nephrotic syndrome generally manifest heavy proteinuria and signs of lipiduria (oval fat bodies, fatty casts) on examination of the urine sediment.

Diabetic nephropathy can be diagnosed on clinical grounds alone in patients presenting with diabetes mellitus of long duration, heavy proteinuria, retinopathy, hypertension, and a consistent urine sediment (i.e., hyaline and granular casts with oval fat bodies or fatty casts in nephrotic subjects). In patients with unusual features such as rapid loss of renal function, red blood cell (RBC) casts, or heavy proteinuria occurring after a short duration of diabetes, it is important to consider the presence of nondiabetic renal disease. Although nondiabetic glomerulopathies account for less than 10% of renal disease in diabetics, this possibility may have important therapeutic and prognostic implications.[26–28] The most commonly encountered nondiabetic renal lesions in diabetic patients are membranous nephropathy, post-infectious glomerulonephritis, minimal change disease, and rapidly progressive glomerulonephritis.[28, 29] Each of these disorders has a clinical course, treatment, and prognosis sufficiently different from diabetic nephropathy to warrant definitive diagnosis with renal biopsy whenever atypical clinical features raise the suspicion of nondiabetic renal disease in a patient with known diabetes.

Treatment

Management of patients with diabetic nephropathy includes general supportive measures such as prevention of fluid overload and congestive heart failure, identification and treatment of urinary tract infection, and ophthalmologic consultation for treatment of retinopathy. As renal function declines, insulin dosages often require downward adjustments and may be only a fraction of initial requirements as the patient approaches ESRD. General management issues relating to patients with the nephrotic syndrome are discussed in Chapter 6.

Although tight control of blood glucose may theoretically prevent or delay the development of diabetic nephropathy, few data are actually available to support this contention. Until recently this lack of clear-cut evidence has stemmed from the inability to "normalize" blood glucose throughout the day and from the difficulty in identifying that portion of the diabetic population at risk for the development of diabetic nephropathy. The recent availability of the insulin pump and home blood glucose monitoring, combined with the finding that microalbuminuria predicts the development of overt nephropathy, has produced some important but preliminary observations. Viberti et al. showed that short-term continuous subcutaneous insulin administration reduced or normalized urinary albumin excretion in patients with diabetes and microalbuminuria.[14] In addition, a recent study comparing two years of continuous subcutaneous insulin to conventional insulin therapy demonstrated that intensive treatment resulted in a reduction of supernormal GFRs to the normal range.[30] By contrast, some workers have found no correlation between glycosylated hemoglobin and declining renal function and have shown that continuous subcutaneous insulin does not influence the course of clinically overt proteinuria.[23, 31] These findings suggest that established nephropathy is resistant to at least short-term intensive insulin treatment but that individuals with incipient disease may benefit from aggressive therapy. Clearly, long-term studies will be required to resolve these issues.

In contrast to the equivocal findings regarding the effects of strict glycemic control on the development and progression of diabetic nephropathy, there is general agreement that effective antihypertensive therapy is beneficial in slowing the decline in renal function. Mogensen demonstrated that reduction of arterial pressure from a mean of 160/103 mm Hg to 144/95 mm Hg decreased the rate of decline of

GFR by 50% (Fig 4–5).[32] Other workers have shown that, in patients with established nephropathy, proteinuria stabilized or decreased with normalization of mean arterial pressure.[31] Thus, treatment of hypertension appears to beneficially influence the course of diabetic nephropathy, possibly by its effects on intraglomerular hemodynamics.[13] Some investigators recommend that diastolic blood pressure be maintained at less than 100 mm Hg as a minimum.[23]

Although the rate at which renal function declines may be modified, progression to ESRD remains inevitable for patients with clinically overt diabetic nephropathy. Survival of diabetics with ESRD is significantly poorer than that of patients with ESRD due to other causes.[33] This is not surprising in view of the diffuse vascular disease associated with longstanding diabetes mellitus. Survival of patients receiving a kidney transplant from a related donor exceeds that of patients undergoing cadaveric transplantation or dialysis. Recent analyses suggest that survival rates in diabetics treated by cadaveric transplantation or dialysis are equivalent.[33] Transplantation is a

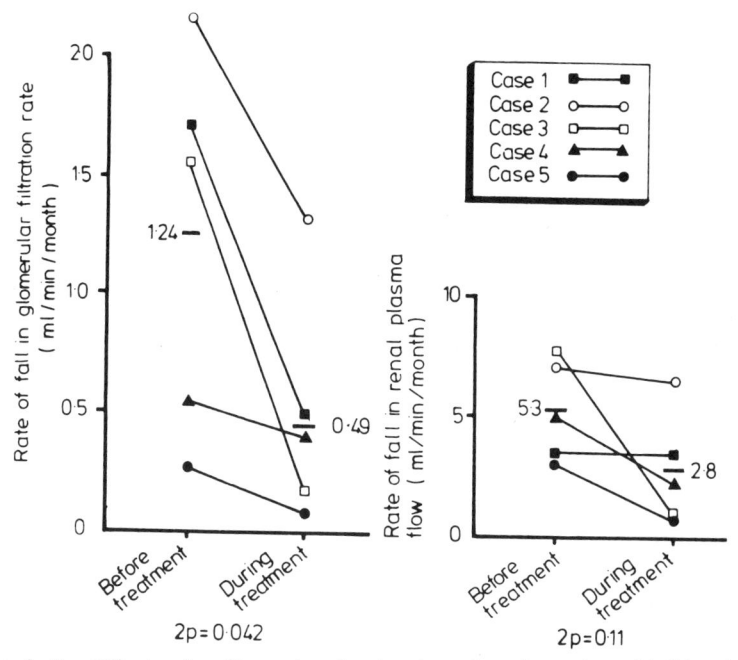

Fig 4–5.—Effects of antihypertensive treatment on the rates of fall in glomerular filtration rate *(left panel)* and renal plasma flow *(right panel)* in five patients with diabetic nephropathy. (Courtesy of Mogensen C.E.: *Br. Med. J.* 285:687, 1982.)

more cost-effective treatment modality than hemodialysis and has the potential for improved patient rehabilitation. However, it is not a panacea. Progression of vascular disease often continues, resulting in substantial morbidity and mortality from cardiovascular complications.[1, 4] Furthermore, recurrent diabetic glomerulosclerosis has been reported in renal allografts.[7, 34] Despite these problems, live, related donor transplantation is the preferred therapeutic approach in suitable candidates. If related donor transplantation is not possible, the choice between cadaveric transplantation and long-term dialysis must be guided by considerations such as patient desires, age, surgical risk, coexistent morbidity, and cost.

Dialysis will usually be required in most diabetics even if transplantation is eventually contemplated. It is important to anticipate the progression of renal failure to plan for construction of vascular access and institution of dialysis. Diabetics frequently require access revision and are generally more symptomatic at any given level of renal function compared to nondiabetics.[2] Consequently, it is our preference to establish vascular access when the GFR reaches 15 ml/minute and to begin dialysis at a GFR of approximately 10 ml/minute. Careful medical management allows reasonable but not ideal rehabilitation. Continuous ambulatory peritoneal dialysis (CAPD) has been used with limited success in diabetics but, in addition to the usual complications of peritonitis and protein-calorie malnutrition, CAPD poses the added burden of further glucose loads. Nevertheless, this is a useful treatment alternative in selected patients, particularly those with repeated failure of vascular access.

SYSTEMIC LUPUS ERYTHEMATOSUS

Epidemiology

Renal involvement is a frequent if not invariable manifestation of systemic lupus erythematosus (SLE) and produces substantial morbidity and mortality. The epidemiologic pattern of lupus nephritis closely parallels that of SLE itself. SLE is six to eight times more prevalent in females than males and much more common in blacks compared to whites. The peak onset of clinically apparent SLE ranges between 10 and 40 years of age.[35] Familial clustering of the disease occurs and recent studies suggest a genetic predisposition to SLE.[36] Clinically evident renal disease is present in two thirds of patients with SLE at the time of initial diagnosis.[36, 37] However, studies based on renal biopsies suggest that virtually all patients have renal histologic abnormalities, irrespective of clinical renal involvement.[37] Renal manifestations of SLE vary from isolated proteinuria to rapidly progressive glomerulonephritis. Nephrotic range proteinuria occurs in over 50% of patients at some time during the disease.

Pathology

The pathologic classification of lupus nephritis has undergone substantial revision during the past decade, reflecting in part an imperfect correlation between histologic abnormalities and clinical course. Recently, attempts have been made to score renal biopsy specimens on the basis of an activity and chronicity index.[36, 38] This scoring system, however, has not achieved widespread popularity to date; a modification of the World Health Organization's classification is still most useful. The WHO system separates lupus nephritis into four basic histologic categories: mesangial, focal proliferative, diffuse proliferative, and membranous lupus nephritis. It should be noted, however, that transitions from one histologic classification to another occur in 15% to 20% of patients with lupus nephritis. In all likelihood this dynamic renal histopathology represents spontaneous alterations in the patient's immunologic status, the effects of immunosuppressive therapy, and multiple other factors.

Mesangial involvement accounts for 15% of all lupus nephritis and is probably the lowest common denominator with regard to histologic abnormalities. It is a frequent histologic finding even in patients without clinically overt renal disease.[37] Using light microscopy, the glomeruli in mesangial lupus nephritis may appear normal, show mild expansion of the mesangial matrix, or exhibit mild mesangial hypercellularity (Fig 4–6,A). Irrespective of light microscopic changes, immunofluorescent studies reveal mesangial deposition of IgG and C3 in the majority of cases; IgA and IgM are seen with lesser frequency.[36, 39] Electron-dense deposits correspond to the positive mesangial immunofluorescence.

Focal proliferative glomerulonephritis is found in approximately 25% of patients with lupus nephritis. This lesion is characterized by a focal (less than 50% of all glomeruli), segmental (some but not all glomerular tufts) endothelial cell proliferation (Figure 4–6,B). An increase in mesangial cells and matrix occurs in about one third of cases.[39] Immune-deposits of IgG, C3, and to a lesser extent IgA and IgM are found throughout the mesangium and along peripheral cap-

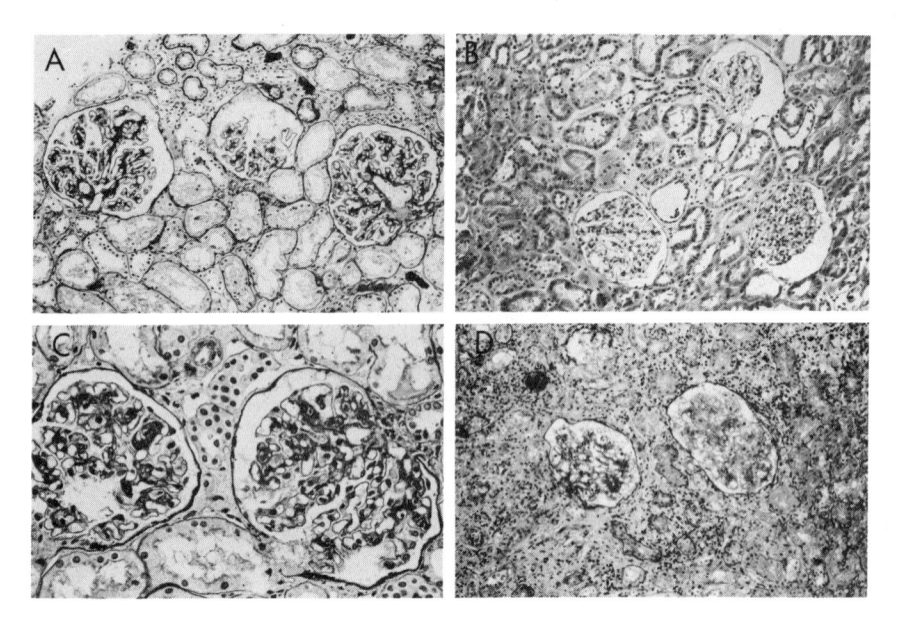

Fig 4–6.—Four basic histologic patterns of lupus nephritis. **A,** periodic acid-Schiff-stained section of mesangial lupus nephritis. The only histologic abnormality is a mild increase in the mesangial matrix. **B,** hematoxylin- and eosin-stained section demonstrating focal proliferative glomerulonephritis. There is a focal segmental increase in endothelial and mesangial cells. **C,** periodic acid-Schiff-stained section of diffuse proliferative lupus nephritis. There is generalized expansion of the mesangial matrix and an increase in both mesangial and endothelial cells. **D,** periodic acid-Schiff-stained section of membranous lupus nephropathy. There is marked expansion of the mesangial matrix, moderate widening of the GBM and no increase in cellularity.

illary loops. Electron microscopy reveals electron-dense deposits in the mesangium and capillary wall. The capillary loop deposits are most prominent in subendothelial portions of the GBM but occasionally are distributed in subepithelial or intramembranous locations as well.

Diffuse proliferative lupus nephritis accounts for 50% of all cases of renal involvement in SLE. By light microscopy this lesion is qualitatively similar but quantitatively more extensive than the focal variety, being characterized by a marked increase in both endothelial and mesangial cells and mesangial matrix in all glomeruli (Fig 4–6,C). Thickening of capillary loops is variable but may be extensive enough to result in a simplified glomerular architecture that resembles idiopathic membranoproliferative glomerulonephritis (MPGN).[36] Some investigators, in fact, consider MPGN as a distinct subset of lupus nephritis; however, because the clinical course of lupus MPGN is indistinguishable from diffuse proliferative glomerulonephritis, this distinction serves no clinically useful purpose. In severe forms of diffuse proliferative nephritis, cellular crescents, tubular atrophy, and glomerular sclerosis indicate an increased risk of progression to ESRD.[40] Immunofluorescent staining is positive for IgG, C3, IgM, and to a lesser extent IgA in a mesangial distribution and in capillary loops. Electron-dense deposits in the mesangium and subendothelial space correspond to the immunofluorescent findings and generally parallel the severity of the light microscopic changes.[39]

Membranous glomerulonephritis occurs in approximately 10% of patients with lupus nephritis and may be histologically indistinguishable from idiopathic membranous glomerulopathy. In membranous lupus nephritis, light microscopic findings vary from mild mesangial expansion and apparently normal capillary loops to a definite increase in mesangial cellularity with clearly thickened capillary walls (Fig 4–6,D). Capillary loops stain for IgG and C3 in a finely granular pattern; IgA and IgM are found infrequently. Electron microscopy discloses the subepithelial electron-dense deposits characteristic of membranous glomerulopathy. In addition, small subendothelial and mesangial deposits may be found in a minority of cases. These latter findings, coupled with an increase in mesangial cellularity, should raise the possibility of membranous lupus nephritis even in the absence of other diagnostic criteria for SLE.[41]

Pathophysiology

The pathophysiology of SLE and lupus nephritis has been investigated extensively.[36] The development of SLE depends on the interaction of genetic factors, gender, and environmental influences. Protean immunologic abnormalities of both B-cell and T-cell function occur in SLE and result in the production of various autoantibodies, most notably antilymphocyte and antinuclear antibodies. Current data suggest that under the proper genetic and environmental circumstances, polyclonal B-cell proliferation results in antilymphocyte antibodies that inhibit suppressor T-cell function. This inhibition of suppressor T lymphocytes causes further unrestrained antibody synthesis. Production of antinuclear antibodies results in the formation of circulating immune-complexes, deposition in various organs, and tissue inflammation.[36]

Renal disease in SLE appears to result from the deposition of DNA-anti-DNA complexes within the kidney; however, not all patients with circulating DNA-anti-DNA complexes develop clinically significant renal disease. Reticuloendothelial function, antibody class, complement fixation, and the size of complexes are just some factors that influence the ability of immune-complexes to produce disease. Complement-fixing, precipitating IgG antibody is most frequently associated with renal disease in SLE.[42-44] Antibody to DNA can be eluted from glomeruli of patients with lupus nephritis, strongly suggesting that DNA-anti-DNA complexes are related etiologically to the renal disease.[45] Mesangial, focal proliferative and diffuse proliferative lupus nephritis may result from the deposition of circulating immune-complexes. However, the histologic similarity between membranous lupus nephritis and idiopathic membranous glomerulopathy suggests that this type of renal disease may result from in situ immune-complex formation.

Clinical Features

Most patients with SLE have clinically apparent renal involvement at the time lupus is first diagnosed. However, histologic evidence of renal disease is present in virtually all patients with SLE regardless of clinical or laboratory findings.[37, 46] Renal manifestations are the dominant feature of SLE in one quarter of patients at the time of initial diagnosis; in 5% of subjects, renal disease antedates all other manifestations of SLE. Extrarenal disease is a frequent accompaniment and includes arthritis, cutaneous lesions, serositis, and hema-

TABLE 4–2.—CLINICAL FEATURES OF LUPUS NEPHRITIS IN 370 PATIENTS*

	MESANGIAL LUPUS NEPHRITIS	FOCAL PROLIFERATIVE LUPUS NEPHRITIS	MEMBRANOUS LUPUS NEPHRITIS	DIFFUSE PROLIFERATIVE LUPUS NEPHRITIS
Percent of total cases	15	25	10	50
Hematuria	30	75	50	75
Proteinuria	75	90	100	95
Hypertension	10	10	25	50
Nephrotic syndrome	0–5	10	70	80
Renal insufficiency at diagnosis	0–5	10	10	75
Progression to ESRD at 5 yrs	0–5	15	10	40
Mortality at 5 yrs	10	20	40	45

*Approximate percentages, from Cameron,[35] Decker,[36] Mahajan,[37] and Baldwin.[39]

tologic abnormalities.[35] In general, there is a rough correlation between extrarenal manifestations, serologic evidence of disease activity, histologic classification, and progression of clinical renal disease. This relation is only approximate, however, and numerous exceptions exist. Nevertheless, it is convenient to discuss the clinical features of lupus nephritis in terms of the underlying histologic lesion.

The salient clinical features of lupus nephritis are summarized in Table 4–2. These data represent an approximation of the percentages of patients in each histologic category demonstrating the indicated sign or symptom. Because clinically occult lupus nephritis has only recently been recognized, these figures undoubtedly overestimate the prevalence of each feature in a given histologic class. Still, they provide clinically useful estimates for the clinician caring for patients with SLE.

Patients with mesangial lupus nephritis have the mildest form of renal involvement; many have no urinary abnormalities when SLE is first diagnosed.[37, 46] Clinically apparent mesangial lupus nephritis is characterized by microscopic hematuria or minimal proteinuria in most patients. Hypertension is rare and the nephrotic syndrome extremely unusual. Few patients progress to renal insufficiency and death is generally related to the extrarenal manifestations of SLE. The development of renal insufficiency or nephrotic range proteinuria in a patient with biopsy proven mesangial nephritis should raise the suspicion of a transition to a histologically more severe variety of lupus nephritis.[39]

Focal proliferative glomerulonephritis accounts for 25% of all cases of lupus nephritis. Proteinuria is found in 90% or more of patients with this lesion and hematuria is frequent. Hypertension, mild renal insufficiency, and the nephrotic syndrome occur in approximately 10% of cases. The extremely favorable prognosis once associated with this lesion probably reflected the inadvertent inclusion of patients with mesangial lupus nephritis. Since the recognition of mesangial nephritis as a distinct entity, investigators have described a greater progression to ESRD and higher mortality rate in focal proliferative lupus nephritis. It is likely that the development of progressive renal insufficiency in patients with the focal lesion signals the histologic evolution to diffuse proliferative glomerulonephritis.

Proteinuria occurs in virtually all patients with membranous lupus nephropathy and ultimately progresses to the nephrotic syndrome in approximately three quarters of cases. Hematuria, hypertension, and mild renal insufficiency at the outset occur with much less frequency.

Rare transitions to diffuse proliferative lupus nephritis have been described. Severe renal insufficiency and ESRD ensue in 10% of cases of membranous nephropathy and are usually associated with persistent heavy proteinuria unresponsive to steroid therapy.[39]

Diffuse proliferative lupus nephritis is the most common and severe form of renal involvement in SLE. Hematuria, hypertension, and varying degrees of renal insufficiency are present in 50% to 75% of patients when renal disease is clinically apparent. Proteinuria occurs in over 90%; about 80% of patients develop the nephrotic syndrome. Considering the prevalence of diffuse proliferative glomerulonephritis and its frequent association with nephrotic range proteinuria, the great majority of patients with SLE and the nephrotic syndrome are likely to have this lesion on a statistical basis alone. Spontaneous histologic transitions of diffuse proliferative lupus nephritis are rare but steroid therapy has been associated with transition to the membranous form. Diffuse proliferative glomerulonephritis is associated with an ominous prognosis in patients with SLE.[38, 40] As many as 40% develop ESRD within five years of diagnosis and the five-year mortality approaches 50%.

Implicit in the above classification scheme is the assumption that knowledge of the precise histologic diagnosis provides important information relevant to prognosis and therapeutic strategy. However, Fries and associates have suggested that classification of lupus nephritis by clinical criteria including serum creatinine, BUN, and total hemolytic complement (CH50) provides as much prognostic information as a limited histologic classification.[47] These findings, together with the obvious overlap among the clinical features of lupus nephritis, have led some investigators to question the utility of renal biopsy in patients with SLE. More recent studies suggest that improved histologic classification according to a chronicity index provides important data with regard to both prognosis and therapy.[38, 48] The value of renal biopsy in lupus nephritis remains controversial. Our preference is to withhold biopsy in patients with minimal urinary abnormalities and essentially normal renal function. We employ steroids to treat extrarenal manifestations, when indicated, and carefully monitor renal function. If we contemplate the addition of cytotoxic therapy to a corticosteroid regimen, we generally advocate biopsy to select those subjects likely to derive maximum benefit (see below).

Even with optimal medical management, a significant number of patients with lupus nephritis ultimately develop ESRD.[49-52] Patients with the specific histologic findings of tubular atrophy, glomerular sclerosis, and cellular crescents have a high likelihood of progressing to chronic renal failure irrespective of their conventional histologic classification.[40] Survival of subjects with ESRD due to lupus nephritis is probably decreased compared to dialysis patients with primary renal diseases,[49, 51] although some reports have shown similar survival in both populations.[50] Morbidity and mortality result largely from infectious complications and poor patency of vascular access. Most workers agree that extrarenal manifestations of SLE decrease markedly with the development of ESRD and institution of maintenance dialysis.[49, 50]

Therapy

Despite extensive clinical trials, there is currently no single uniformly accepted approach to the treatment of lupus nephritis. Optimal therapeutic strategies remain a subject of controversy for several reasons. First, although there is a general correlation between conventional renal histologic classification and development of renal insufficiency, there are no easily measurable serologic parameters that reliably predict the progression of renal disease. Moreover, urinary abnormalities correlate poorly with underlying histopathology and do not predict ultimate outcome.[37, 46] Except for examination of sequential renal biopsy specimens, there are few readily determined parameters to follow as an index of the activity or progression of renal disease. Finally, subclinical histologic transitions occur that are not reflected in alterations in BUN, serum creatinine, or urinary protein excretion.

Our approach to the management of lupus nephritis (Fig 4–7) combines measurement of serologic activity, estimates of renal function, determinations of urinary protein excretion, and judicious use of renal biopsy to guide therapeutic decisions. In nonazotemic patients with minimal urinary abnormalities (i.e., hematuria, proteinuria less than 3.0 gm) and a normal CH50, oral corticosteroid therapy is employed as needed to treat the extrarenal manifestations of SLE. For nonazotemic patients with minimal urinary abnormalities and hypocomplementemia, we recommend intravenous methylprednisolone in a dose of 1 gm daily for 3 days, followed by moderate doses of prednisone (0.5 mg/kg/day) for 6 to 8 weeks. If the CH50 returns to normal, the dose of prednisone is tapered and maintained at the lowest dose compatible with a normal serum complement. Recent work suggests that prolonged normalization of CH50 is associated with both stable renal histology and serum creatinine levels.[53] Pulse methyl-

Minimal urinary abnormalities and creatinine <1.4 mg/dl

Treat with steroids depending on extra renal disease

- Normal CH50
- Decreased CH50 → Methylprednisolone 1 gram daily × 3 then Prednisone 0.5 mg/kg/day × 6–8 weeks.
  - Normal CH50
  - Decreased CH50 → Taper & discontinue steroids. Monitor creatinine, protein excretion and extra renal disease
  - Taper dose and maintain at lowest dose that normalizes CH_{50}.

Creatinine >1.4 mg/dl, Protein excretion >3 grams or both.

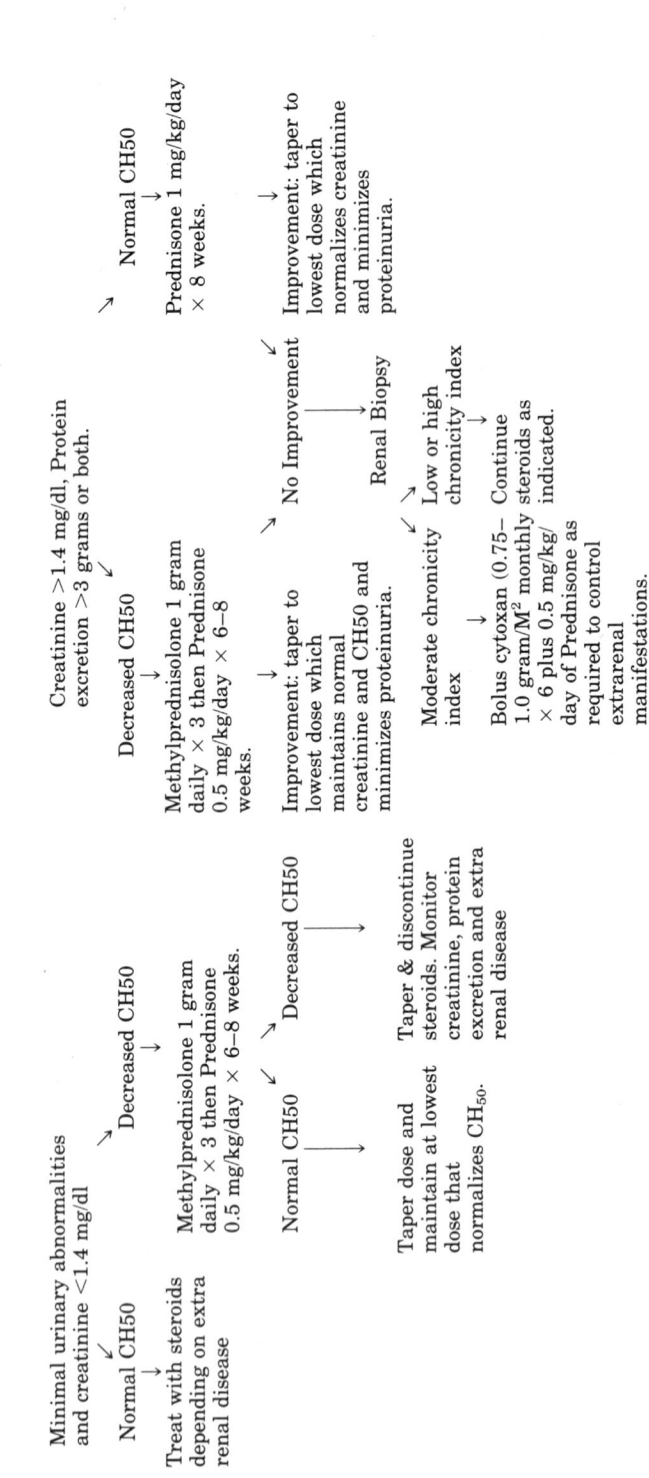

- Normal CH50 → Prednisone 1 mg/kg/day × 8 weeks.
  - Improvement: taper to lowest dose which normalizes creatinine and minimizes proteinuria.
- Decreased CH50 → Methylprednisolone 1 gram daily × 3 then Prednisone 0.5 mg/kg/day × 6–8 weeks.
  - Improvement: taper to lowest dose which maintains normal creatinine and CH50 and minimizes proteinuria.
  - No Improvement → Renal Biopsy
    - Low or high chronicity index → Continue steroids as indicated.
    - Moderate chronicity index → Bolus cytoxan (0.75–1.0 gram/M² monthly × 6 plus 0.5 mg/kg/day of Prednisone as required to control extrarenal manifestations.

Fig 4–7.—Treatment strategy for the management of lupus nephritis.

prednisolone allows the subsequent use of lower doses of oral corticosteroid and is particularly effective in hypocomplementemic lupus nephritis.[54] Oral prednisone in a dose of 1 mg/kg/day is probably equally effective. We taper and eventually discontinue steroids in patients who fail to normalize serum complement levels with this regimen. However, these patients require close monitoring of urinary protein excretion and renal function. Deterioration of renal function or development of the nephrotic syndrome usually warrants more aggressive steroid therapy or cytotoxic drug administration.

Patients with elevated serum creatinine levels, nephrotic syndrome, or both, are at high risk to develop ESRD on clinical grounds alone.[38] Consequently, these patients should receive corticosteroid therapy irrespective of serum complement levels. It is our preference to treat hypocomplementemic patients with pulse methylprednisolone as previously described, reserving high dose oral prednisone (1 mg/kg/day) for patients with normal CH50 levels. In both groups, further adjustment of steroid dosage is guided primarily by changes in serum creatinine and protein excretion. Patients with clinically severe lupus nephritis, unresponsive to either of these steroid regimens, are candidates for cytotoxic drug therapy.

Although early studies employing conventional histologic criteria showed little or no benefit from either oral azathioprine or cyclophosphamide,[35, 36] recent investigations suggest substantial benefit when subjects are classified on the basis of chronic histologic changes. Utilizing a chronicity index based on the degree of glomerular sclerosis, fibrous crescents, tubular atrophy, and interstitial fibrosis, investigators at the National Institutes of Health (NIH) found stabilization of both renal function and histology in patients treated with oral or intravenous cytotoxic drugs.[48, 55] Considering the potential hazards of long-term cytotoxic drug administration, including sterility, neoplasia, leukopenia, and cystitis, it is important to select the least toxic treatment regimen for subjects who are most likely to benefit from such therapy.[56-58] We perform renal biopsy in all patients who are being considered for cytotoxic drug therapy. Patients who demonstrate a moderate chronicity index appear to benefit most from cytotoxic therapy in addition to steroids compared to conventional steroid regimens alone.[48] By contrast, patients with low or high chronicity indices derive no obvious benefit from cytotoxic treatment. Prolonged oral cyclophosphamide therapy is associated with an unacceptably high incidence of adverse reactions[56-58] and has been abandoned in favor of oral azathioprine or intermittent intravenous cyclophosphamide. Both appear equally effective, but we prefer the latter based on less toxicity and the theoretical advantages of intermittent as opposed to continuous immunosuppression.[58, 60] Plasmapharesis combined with corticosteroid and cytotoxic drug therapy has produced inconsistent preliminary results in patients with diffuse proliferative glomerulonephritis, and its role in the treatment of lupus nephritis remains to be determined.

Dialysis and transplantation are acceptable modes of therapy for patients who progress to chronic renal failure in spite of all therapeutic interventions. Most studies have shown that clinical and serologic manifestations of extrarenal SLE improve during long-term hemodialysis despite withdrawal of immunosuppressive drugs.[49, 51] It is important to note that approximately one third of all patients eventually regain sufficient renal function to discontinue dialysis,[51, 52] a phenomenon most commonly observed in the subgroup of lupus patients with rapidly progressive glomerulonephritis. Patients with lupus nephritis of less than two years duration who rapidly progress to "end-stage" renal disease should probably be treated with moderate doses of corticosteroids for at least two months after institution of dialysis until the irreversibility of their renal failure has been reasonably established. Patients with chronic renal failure due to lupus nephritis are candidates for transplantation based on the same criteria as the general ESRD population. Renal transplantation has been performed successfully in patients with SLE; the recurrence rate of lupus nephritis in allografts is about 10%.[61]

AMYLOIDOSIS

Epidemiology

Amyloidosis is a disease complex resulting from the deposition of a variety of proteins that share a characteristic beta-pleated sheet structure and common tinctoral properties. Focal accumulations of amyloid are frequently found in elderly subjects at postmortem examination but rarely result in organ dysfunction.[62, 63] By contrast, extensive amyloid deposits in various organs cause significant morbidity and mortality in primary amyloidosis, multiple myeloma, heredofamilial amyloid, and chronic inflammatory or neoplastic disorders. Primary amyloidosis has a peak incidence in the seventh decade and males outnumber females. Amyloidosis may also complicate between 5% to 11% of cases of rheumatoid arthritis and 6% to 15% of cases of multiple myeloma.[63] Even though systemic amyloidosis is a rare disorder, it accounts for 5% to 10% of all cases of the nephrotic syndrome in adults.

Pathology

Routine light microscopy may suggest the presence of amyloid but definitive diagnosis of amyloidosis requires special stains, such as crystal violet or Congo red, or electron microscopy. When stained with Congo red and examined under polarized light, amyloid proteins exhibit a characteristic emerald green birefringence. Electron microscopic examination of amyloid deposits demonstrates a weblike network of linear nonbranching fibrils approximately 7.5 to 10 nm in diameter.[63]

In systemic amyloidosis, amyloid deposits can be identified in multiple organs including liver, heart, skin, the gastrointestinal tract, and kidney. Histologic examination of renal tissue reveals a spectrum of changes depending on the extent of involvement. Although amyloid deposition occurs in the renal blood vessels and interstitium, glomerular amyloid accumulation accounts for the heavy proteinuria. Glomerular abnormalities on light microscopy range from a mild expansion of the mesangial matrix to thickening of the GBM and mesangial nodule formation reminiscent of diabetic glomerulosclerosis (Fig 4–8,A). With hematoxylin and eosin, these deposits assume a pale, amorphous, waxy appearance; metachromatic reactions with crystal violet or characteristic staining with Congo red identify the deposits as amyloid. Immunofluorescent staining is generally negative in amyloidosis. Electron microscopic examination of renal tissue reveals the characteristic fibrillar structure of amyloid in glomeruli and in involved areas of the interstitium and blood vessels (Fig 4–8,B).

Pathophysiology

There are four major categories of systemic amyloidosis and at least six different proteins associated with amyloid formation. A limited classification listing diseases and their major amyloid fibril component is shown in Table 4–3. Localized amyloid deposition occurs in senile cardiac amyloid (AS protein) and in endocrine-related amyloid (AE protein) but is not associated with systemic manifestations or renal involvement.

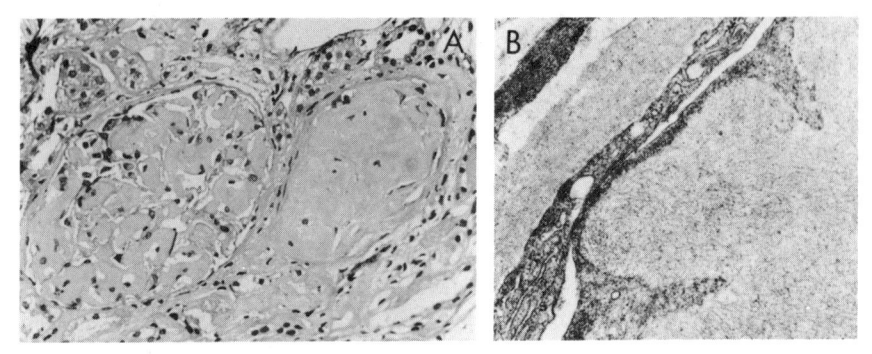

Fig 4–8.—Renal histology in systemic amyloidosis. **A,** light micrograph depicting mesangial nodules. **B,** electron micrograph illustrating weblike amyloid fibrils within the mesangium.

In recent years, the pathogenesis of the systemic amyloidoses has been studied carefully.[63-65] Formation of amyloid protein results from the in vivo proteolytic cleavage of precursor molecules. Both the amyloid of primary amyloidosis and that associated with multiple myeloma or other plasma cell dyscrasias appears to be derived from the variable region of immunoglobulin light chains (AL protein). Durie and co-workers have shown that myeloma cells in culture synthesize Bence Jones proteins; these proteins are processed by associated macrophages with subsequent secretion of amyloid.[65] The major amyloid fibril proteins in patients with secondary amyloidosis or familial Mediterranean fever have a common N-terminal sequence of nine amino acids.[63] This fibril, amyloid A protein (AA), has been identified in several inflammatory and neoplastic disorders associated with secondary amyloidosis.[63-69] AA protein is apparently derived from a serum component, SAA, an acute phase reactant. Increased circulating levels of SAA have been demonstrated in some malignancies, especially renal cell carcinoma, in other forms of secondary amyloidosis,

TABLE 4–3.—CLASSIFICATION OF THE AMYLOIDOSES

CLASSIFICATION	ASSOCIATED DISEASE	FIBRIL PROTEIN
Primary amyloidosis	None	AL
Myeloma associated	Multiple myeloma	AL
Secondary	Chronic inflammatory or suppurative conditions (e.g., rheumatoid arthritis, tuberculosis, Hodgkin's disease)	AA
Heredofamilial	Familial Mediterranean fever	AA

and in familial Mediterranean fever.[69] Abnormal processing of SAA by macrophages probably results in AA fibril formation in a manner analogous to the production of AL fibrils.[63]

Clinical Features

The clinical manifestations of the amyloidoses depend chiefly on the underlying cause of amyloid deposition and whether cardiac or renal involvement is dominant. Monoclonal serum or urinary proteins (whole immunoglobulins, or light chains, or both) are present in virtually all cases of primary amyloidosis. Lambda light chains predominate over kappa light chains in a ratio of 2:1.[63] Extrarenal manifestations of primary amyloidosis include peripheral neuropathy, restrictive cardiomyopathy, purpura, polyarthopathy, and macroglossia.[63, 67, 70] Hepatic enlargement may be prominent, but liver function is usually well preserved. In myeloma-associated amyloid, similar extrarenal features occur in addition to the manifestations of myeloma itself.

Secondary or reactive amyloidosis is associated with chronic inflammatory conditions such as rheumatoid arthritis, osteomyelitis, tuberculosis, systemic lupus erythematosus, regional ileitis, bronchiectasis and familial Mediterranean fever. In addition, neoplastic diseases, most notably renal cell carcinoma and Hodgkin's disease, have been linked to the development of amyloidosis of the AA type.[69] Cardinal features of secondary amyloidosis include progressive hepatosplenomegaly and heavy proteinuria. The occurrence of reactive amyloidosis is associated with substantially reduced survival compared to patients with similar disorders who do not develop amyloidosis.[63]

Proteinuria, occurring in over 90% of cases, may provide a clue to the development of amyloidosis in patients with predisposing disease. The nephrotic syndrome develops in only 30% of patients with primary amyloidosis and in about 50% of subjects with reactive amyloid.[70] Orthostatic hypotension attributable to hypoalbuminemia, autonomic neuropathy, and cardiac involvement is not uncommon; consequently, hypertension is unusual even in patients with ESRD.[71] Tubulointerstitial disease is occasionally the predominant renal disorder in amyloidosis and may be manifest by isolated renal tubular acidosis or the Fanconi syndrome.

The diagnosis of amyloidosis may be suspected under the appropriate clinical circumstances but requires histologic confirmation. Demonstration of amyloid by subcutaneous fat pad aspiration or rectal biopsy in proteinuric patients is usually sufficient to establish the diagnosis of renal amyloidosis and precludes the need for kidney biopsy. Both are high-yield, low morbidity procedures and are positive in approximately 80% to 85% of patients.[63] We reserve renal biopsy for patients in whom these less risky procedures are nondiagnostic or for cases in which an additional cause of the secondary nephrotic syndrome (e.g., diabetes, SLE) may complicate the clinical picture.

Treatment

The therapeutic approach to renal amyloidosis should include a search for underlying disorders associated with reactive amyloidosis. Occasionally, identification and treatment of associated diseases results in remission of the amyloidosis.[63] However, the prognosis is grim in most patients with secondary amyloidosis and those with primary or myeloma-related amyloid; survival is less than two years from the time of diagnosis in the majority of cases. Unfortunately, there are no long-term controlled clinical trials that clearly demonstrate the efficacy of any therapeutic regimen. Nevertheless, small series and isolated case reports suggest that potentially effective treatments are available.[63, 72-75] Given the poor prognosis of amyloidosis, a therapeutic trial may be warranted even in the absence of conclusive studies.

Because primary amyloidosis is an immunocyte disorder, it seems logical that cytotoxic therapy directed at an abnormal clone of plasma cells might prove beneficial. In this regard, several studies have reported improvement or resolution of primary amyloidosis during treatment with prednisone and an alkylating agent.[63, 72, 73] Ravid and co-workers reported that colchicine in a daily dose of 1.0 to 1.5 mg resulted in resolution of the nephrotic syndrome and modest improvement in GFR in a single patient with primary amyloidosis and three with familial Mediterranean fever.[74] The same group of investigators have noted preliminary success treating secondary amyloid due to a variety of disorders with dimethylsulfoxide (DMSO), a denaturing agent effective in experimental amyloidosis.[75] Based on these encouraging but preliminary results, it would seem reasonable to treat patients with primary amyloidosis with monthly courses of prednisone and an alkylating agent. Patients with amyloid due to familial Mediterranean fever should be treated with colchicine; whereas those with secondary amyloid, refractory to eradication of the underlying disorder, might be considered for a trial of DMSO.

Edema formation is common in amyloidosis and results both from hypoalbuminemia consequent to the nephrotic syndrome and cardiac failure. As a rule, edematous patients should be treated cautiously with diuretics because of their propensity to develop orthostatic hypotension. Patients with amyloid cardiomyopathy are highly sensitive to the cardiotoxic effects of digitalis, perhaps because of enhanced binding of digitalis to amyloid fibrils in the myocardium. Hemodialysis and transplantation have been employed to treat ESRD in patients with amyloidosis. Patients without significant cardiac involvement experience a morbidity and mortality similar to that of subjects undergoing dialysis because of primary renal disease.[71] Experience is limited with regard to the long-term results of transplantation. Although recurrence of amyloid in the allograft has been described, renal functional deterioration is rare.[76]

DRUGS AND TOXINS

The kidney is uniquely sensitive to toxic injury because of its large blood flow, high oxygen consumption, and its capacity to concentrate solutes. With the rapid increase in the number of newer pharmacologic agents, drugs are frequently implicated in the development of renal disease. Acute or chronic renal failure and fluid and electrolyte disturbances are the most common drug-related renal syndromes.[77, 78] However, nephrotic range proteinuria is an often overlooked but potentially reversible consequence of drug therapy, especially with some of the newer therapeutic agents. Table 4–4 lists a number of drugs that have been linked to the development of the nephrotic syndrome. Many have been reported anecdotally, but others have been implicated sufficiently to suggest a clear etiologic relationship. We limit the following discussion to those agents most frequently associated with the development of heavy proteinuria.

Gold

A large body of evidence suggests that chrysotherapy may be nephrotoxic.[79–83] Proteinuria occurs with greater frequency in patients with rheumatoid arthritis treated with injectable gold salts than in those treated with a placebo. Overall, approximately 3% to 4% of subjects develop proteinuria during gold therapy; of these, one quarter (i.e., less than 1% of all patients receiving gold) develop heavy proteinuria.[83] Renal tissue from proteinuric patients treated with gold

TABLE 4–4.—Drugs Associated With the
Nephrotic Syndrome

Heavy Metals	Oral Hypoglycemics
Gold	Chlorpropamide
Mercury	Tolbutamide
Anticonvulsants	*Miscellaneous*
Trimethadione	Penicillamine
Paramethadione	Captopril
Nonsteroidal Anti-Inflammatory	"Street" heroin
Drugs	Cimetidine
Fenoprofen	Lithium
Naproxen	Probenecid
Tolmetin	Dapsone
Zomepirac	Perchlorate
Indomethacin	
Sulindac	

exhibits the histologic changes of classical membranous glomerulopathy in over 70% of cases.[79, 80] A significant minority of patients exhibit minimal glomerular changes or nonspecific proliferative lesions.

Not all investigators agree that chrysotherapy is a cause of membranous nephropathy. Samuels and co-workers studied 90 patients with membranous glomerulopathy and found that 8 patients had coexistent rheumatoid arthritis. In only four of the eight could gold treatment be linked to the development of the renal lesion.[81] These workers postulated that gold salts might exacerbate a clinically occult renal lesion, but concluded that there was little evidence to support a causative relation between chrysotherapy and membranous nephropathy. Nevertheless, the infrequent occurrence of membranous glomerulopathy in patients with rheumatoid arthritis not treated with gold suggests that the link between the two is not merely a chance association.

The mechanism by which gold salts induce proteinuria is poorly understood. Because gold can be demonstrated in proximal tubular cells by ultrastructural examination, some workers have theorized that gold-induced proximal tubular injury results in the release of renal tubular epithelial antigen. This previously sequestered autoantigen might become implanted in the GBM with subsequent in situ immune-complex formation (see Chapter 2).[80] A similar sequence of events has been suggested to account for the glomerular lesions in sickle cell nephropathy and some cases of idiopathic membranous glomerulopathy.[84, 85] Another possible, but untested, hypothesis suggests that gold causes aggregation of circulating immunoglobulins that subsequently deposit in the GBM.[80]

Whatever the pathogenetic mechanism, the occurrence of proteinuria and the nephrotic syndrome is more frequent with parenteral gold therapy than with oral gold treatment.[82, 83] Proteinuria may develop after one week to six years of gold therapy, suggesting an idiosyncratic reaction rather than a dose related nephrotoxic effect. When increasing proteinuria or the nephrotic syndrome occurs in patients receiving gold, chrysotherapy should be discontinued. In over 80%, proteinuria resolves within one year following cessation of gold therapy.[79, 83] In one study, short-term rechallenge with gold did not result in relapse in seven of eight previously proteinuric patients.[83] Given the natural history of gold nephropathy after chrysotherapy is discontinued, steroid treatment does not appear warranted.

Nonsteroidal Anti-inflammatory Drugs

Nonsteroidal anti-inflammatory drugs (NSAIDs) are associated with a number of renal syndromes including papillary necrosis, acute renal failure and hyporeninemic hypoaldosteronism. These disorders are probably a direct extension of the action of NSAIDs to inhibit fatty acid cyclo-oxygenase, and occur under conditions in which renal blood flow, GFR, or renin secretion are unusually prostaglandin-dependent (e.g., congestive heart failure, hepatic cirrhosis, chronic renal failure, etc.). In recent years, however, there has been increasing recognition that a variety of NSAIDs may also cause a syndrome of nephrotic range proteinuria and interstitial nephritis.[86–91] This unusual disorder has been described most frequently in association with fenoprofen but also occurs with other NSAIDs (Table 4–4). Heavy proteinuria and variable renal insufficiency develop within 2 weeks to 18 months of NSAID therapy. Urinary protein excretion ranges from 3.5 to over 20 gm per day and renal function may be normal or severely decreased.[86–89, 91] Peripheral eosinophilia, fever, and eosinophiluria are generally absent.[90] In reported cases, renal biopsy has revealed the unusual histologic findings of minimal change glomerular disease and acute interstitial nephritis. Light microscopy demonstrates normal glomerular architecture and an intense mononuclear interstitial infiltrate. Immunofluorescent staining is negative and electron microscopy shows only effacement of epithelial foot processes.

The pathogenesis of this syndrome is unknown. Recent studies utilizing monoclonal antibodies indicate that 75% to 80% of the mononuclear interstitial infiltrate is composed of T lymphocytes.[89, 91] Some workers have theorized that inhibition of cyclo-oxygenase shunts arachidonic acid through the lipoxygenase pathway with subsequent production of mediators of inflammation.[90]

The development of heavy proteinuria, with or without renal insufficiency, in a patient treated with a NSAID should prompt discontinuation of the drug. Although isolated reports suggest a role for corticosteroid administration, most cases have resolved with elimination of the offending agent.[91] In patients with severe renal insufficiency, however, steroids may hasten recovery and reduce the need for dialysis.[87]

Captopril

Proteinuria develops in approximately 1% of patients treated with captopril; nephrotic range proteinuria develops in about 0.3%.[92, 93] Renal biopsy in patients with heavy proteinuria usually reveals findings typical of membranous glomerulopathy. The clinical and histologic similarity between the renal lesions in captopril-treated subjects and the membranous nephropathy due to gold or penicillamine therapy (see below) has led some workers to speculate that captopril can induce an immune-complex nephropathy.[92, 94] Interpretation of available data has been difficult because many early studies included patients with preexisting renal disease or clinically detectable proteinuria. Nevertheless, some workers have shown that, in carefully selected hypertensive patients without evidence of preexisting renal parenchymal disease, administration of captopril results in the development of clinically occult membranous nephropathy in as many as 10%.[94] Although heavy proteinuria occurs most frequently during captopril therapy in subjects with underlying renal disease, there are well-documented instances of nephrotic range proteinuria and membranous nephropathy developing de novo.

The nephrotic syndrome may occur from 3 to 12 months after the institution of captopril. Discontinuation of the drug has resulted in a reduction or elimination of the proteinuria in most cases. However, repeat biopsy has revealed persistence of membranous glomerulopathy for as long as 12 months.[93, 95] The development of significant proteinuria or the nephrotic syndrome during captopril therapy is an indication for discontinuation of the drug. Renal biopsy is usually not warranted unless proteinuria persists or increases; corticosteroids are of no proven benefit.

Heroin

Parenteral drug abuse increases the risk of developing several renal lesions. Glomerulopathies can result from infective endocarditis, chronic HB_sAg antigenemia or amyloidosis.[96] Although the relation of the former lesions to narcotic addiction is generally accepted, the existence of a specific "heroin nephropathy," characterized by the nephrotic syndrome and progressive glomerulosclerosis, has been controversial.[97-100] Rao and co-workers studied 14 heroin addicts with proteinuria; 12 had nephrotic range proteinuria and 11 demonstrated focal glomerulosclerosis on renal biopsy specimens.[97] These investigators suggested that the focal glomerulosclerosis was related etiologically to intravenous heroin abuse. Other workers have detected no substantial difference in the frequency of renal lesions between narcotic addicts and an age-matched control population, and have concluded that no single lesion is consistently associated with narcotic use.[98] Nevertheless, clinicopathologic and epidemiologic studies have shown that heroin-associated nephropathy is a major cause of ESRD in the United States.[99,100] In one survey of metropolitan dialysis units, heroin nephropathy accounted for 11% of all cases of ESRD.[100] The disease is ten times more common in blacks than whites and affects males more frequently than females, but these characteristics may simply reflect the composition of the addict population.

In narcotic addicts, the nephrotic syndrome is most often associated with a renal lesion that resembles idiopathic focal glomerulosclerosis. Light microscopic examination of renal biopsy specimens reveals a variable degree of interstitial nephritis and focal segmental glomerulosclerosis. The sclerotic lesions range from a focal segmental distribution to complete glomerular fibrosis.[97,99] Immunofluorescent staining demonstrates two major patterns; most stain for IgM and C3 in a granular segmental distribution, whereas a significant number reveal linear deposition of IgG along the GBM. This latter finding probably represents nonspecific trapping of IgG similar to that found in diabetic nephropathy. Electron microscopy confirms the light microscopic findings and, notably, fails to reveal evidence of electron-dense deposits.[99]

The pathogenesis of heroin nephropathy is unknown. Some investigators speculate that the lesions result from the injection of adulterants used to dilute the heroin, but firm proof is lacking.[97,99] Whatever the precise etiology, the clinical course of heroin nephropathy is characteristic. Proteinuria, with the full-blown nephrotic syndrome in approximately 50% of patients, develops after several months to years of intravenous narcotic abuse. Renal insufficiency is established in over one half at initial presentation and hypertension is frequent. Approximately two thirds follow an inexorable progression to ESRD over eight months to four years from the onset.[97, 99] There is no specific treatment for heroin nephropathy. The usual therapeutic modalities for ESRD, including hemodialysis, transplantation, and CAPD, should be considered in patients who develop chronic renal failure. If narcotic abuse is avoided after transplantation, this form of focal glomerulosclerosis does not recur in the renal allograft.

Penicillamine

Administration of penicillamine to patients with rheumatoid arthritis, scleroderma, cystinuria, or Wilson's disease is associated with proteinuria in about 10% of cases.[101, 102] There is no clear relationship between either the daily dose or the total cumulative dose and the development of proteinuria. This lack of dose-related nephrotoxicity is reminiscent of gold nephropathy and suggests an idiosyncratic reaction.[101] Proteinuria may occur from four months to five years after institution of penicillamine therapy.

The renal lesion related to penicillamine is usually indistinguishable from idiopathic membranous glomerulopathy.[101] Light microscopy, however, generally reveals only minimal changes; the thickened capillary loops and expansion of mesangial matrix characteristic of advanced membranous nephropathy are frequently absent. Nevertheless, immunofluorescent staining shows IgG and C3 in a finely granular pattern along the peripheral capillary loops, and electron microscopy confirms the presence of subepithelial electron-dense deposits. These consistent histologic findings are observed irrespective of the degree of proteinuria.[101]

The pathogenesis of penicillamine-induced proteinuria is unknown. From 30% to 70% of patients who develop proteinuria progress to the nephrotic syndrome. Penicillamine nephropathy is usually self-limited and resolves with discontinuation of the drug. However, proteinuria and histologic changes may persist for as long as two years after cessation of therapy.[101] Renal insufficiency rarely develops with penicillamine nephropathy, even in patients who develop heavy proteinuria. Therefore, the decision to continue penicillamine in a patient who develops proteinuria or the nephrotic syndrome must be based on a careful assessment of risk versus potential benefit. In patients with a disabling underlying disease, penicillamine might be continued unless symptomatic nephrotic syndrome or renal insufficiency supervene.

Miscellaneous

Heavy proteinuria or the frank nephrotic syndrome has been associated with a number of other therapeutic agents (Table 4–4).[77, 78, 103–105] A spectrum of abnormalities ranging from minimal change disease to proliferative glomerulonephritis has been described. The wide range of histologic lesions accompanying these drug-induced nephrotic syndromes likely reflects a multiplicity of pathogenetic mechanisms. In the vast majority of cases, the nephrotic syndrome resolves with discontinuation of the offending drug.

MALIGNANCY

A large body of evidence supports a link between neoplasia and glomerular disease.[106–108] Glomerulopathies, frequently presenting as nephrotic range proteinuria, have been described in association with carcinomas, Hodgkin's disease, non-Hodgkin's lymphomas, leukemia, and multiple myeloma. An etiologic relationship between cancer and the nephrotic syndrome is supported by several lines of evidence. In 1966, Lee and co-workers reported that 11% of 101 patients with the nephrotic syndrome either had, or developed, a carcinoma.[109] A prospective study by Row and colleagues found 6 cases of malignancy in 77 patients with membranous nephropathy.[109] These and other reports suggest that the incidence of cancer is between 5% and 10% in subjects with the nephrotic syndrome. Numerous investigators have documented a close temporal association between the onset of heavy proteinuria and the diagnosis of cancer. In several instances, successful therapy or excision of the tumor has resulted in clinical and histologic remission of the associated glomerulopathy. Tumor antigens or tumor specific antibodies have been detected in the GBM in a number of reported cases. Taken together, these data provide strong support for a causal relationship between neoplasia and glomerular disease.

In patients with the nephrotic syndrome associated with malignancy, the renal histopathology is closely related to the underlying neoplastic lesion (Table 4–5).[107, 108, 110] Approximately 70% of cases of the nephrotic syndrome in patients with carcinoma are associated with membranous glomerulopathy; the remainder are due to crescentic glomerulonephritis, MPGN, minimal change disease (MCD), or miscellaneous proliferative lesions. Bronchogenic carcinoma accounts for over one third of cancers associated with the nephrotic syndrome, followed in frequency by carcinoma of the colon, kidney, breast, stomach, and pancreas. Before the advent of effective chemotherapy, amyloidosis was the most common cause of heavy proteinuria in patients with Hodgkin's disease. Recent reports and comprehensive reviews, however, suggest that MCD is the most frequent renal lesion in this disorder.[107, 108, 110, 111] Membranous glomerulopathy and various proliferative lesions account for the remaining cases. The nephrotic syndrome has been reported less often in the non-Hodgkin's lymphomas and leukemias; the total number of cases is less than 25 and the lesions appear equally divided among the various histopathologic classifications (Table 4–5).

The pathogenesis of the glomerulopathies related to neoplasia has

TABLE 4–5.—GLOMERULAR PATHOLOGY ASSOCIATED WITH NEOPLASIA

NEOPLASTIC LESION	RENAL PATHOLOGY	% OF CASES*
Carcinoma	Membranous glomerulopathy	70
	Crescentic proliferative	13
	Membranoproliferative	8
	Minimal change	4
	Other†	5
	Total	**100**
Hodgkin's disease	Minimal change	60
	Amyloid	15
	Membranous glomerulopathy	8
	Other†	17
	Total	**100**
Non-Hodgkin's lymphoma	Minimal change	25
	Membranous glomerulopathy	25
	Membranoproliferative	15
	Other†	35
	Total	**100**
Leukemia	Membranous glomerulopathy	25
	Membranoproliferative	15
	Minimal change	10
	Other†	50
	Total	**100**

*Percentages are approximations derived from a review of data.[106–116]
†Includes indeterminate proliferative lesions, mesangial proliferative glomerulonephritis, crescentic glomerulonephritis, and amyloid. Each accounts for less than 10% of the total.

been studied extensively but remains incompletely understood. The most plausible hypothesis accounting for the strong association between carcinoma and membranous nephropathy suggests that tumor antigen, autologous non-tumor antigen, or re-expressed fetal antigens are planted in the GBM, promoting in situ immune-complex formation (see Chapter 2). In this regard, a number of investigators have identified antigen-antibody systems related to tumor specific antigens, renal tubular epithelial antigens, or carcinoembryonic antigen in patients with carcinoma and the nephrotic syndrome,[107, 110, 112–114] By contrast, the pathogenetic link between Hodgkin's disease and MCD is less apparent. Since Hodgkin's disease is a disorder of T lymphocytes, some authors have speculated that abnormal T-cell function with increased lymphokine production could directly alter glomerular permselectivity [111]; however, direct experimental proof is lacking.[112] The possible role of viral antigens in the development of the nephrotic syndrome related to neoplasia has received support from experimental models but requires further clarification in humans.

The relationship between onset of the nephrotic syndrome and diagnosis of malignancy is variable. In the majority of cases, with the notable exception of amyloidosis, heavy proteinuria occurs within one year of the diagnosis of neoplasia. In an exhaustive review of the literature, Eagen and Lewis found that in 80% of cases, the nephrotic syndrome developed in the preceding year or simultaneously with the diagnosis of carcinoma.[107] By contrast, the nephrotic syndrome rarely precedes the diagnosis of Hodgkin's disease; 90% of cases occur with the onset of the disease or during the year following diagnosis. The average age of patients with carcinoma and the nephrotic syndrome is 60. Not surprisingly, prognosis is poor with a median survival of approximately 12 months, usually paralleling the prognosis of the underlying neoplasm. On a number of occasions, however, successful treatment of the neoplasm has been associated with remission of the nephrotic syndrome (Fig 4–9).[107, 108, 110, 115, 116] The prognosis for patients with the nephrotic syndrome related to Hodgkin's disease is much better. Effective chemotherapy or radiotherapy has resulted in complete remission of the nephrotic syndrome due to MCD in more than 95% of reported cases.[110] Further, relapses of MCD linked to recurrences of Hodgkin's disease have been equally responsive to subsequent treatment. Therapy is less successful in inducing remissions of the nephrotic syndrome when other glomerulopathies complicate Hodgkin's disease.

The association between malignancy and the nephrotic syndrome raises two important management issues. The first relates to the ex-

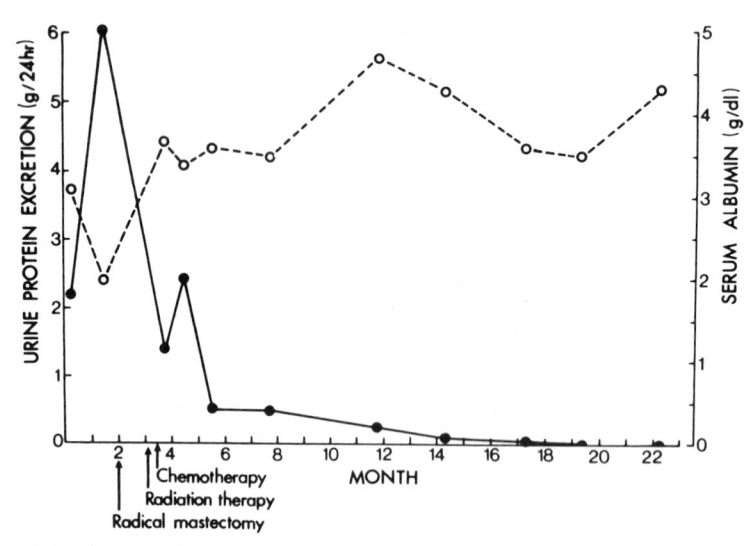

Fig 4–9.—Twenty-four hour urine protein excretion *(closed circles)* and serum albumin concentration *(open circles)* before and after mastectomy, radiation, and chemotherapy in a patient with breast cancer and nephrotic syndrome. (Courtesy of Barton C.H., et al.: *Am. J. Med.* 68:309, 1980.)

tent to which patients with the nephrotic syndrome should be evaluated for an occult neoplasm; the second addresses the role of renal biopsy in subjects with a known malignancy who develop heavy proteinuria. We favor a limited evaluation for occult malignancy in adults over 40 years of age with membranous glomerulopathy. Initial studies should include a physical examination, complete blood count, chest x-ray, and examination of the stool for occult blood (see Chapter 6). Adult patients with presumed idiopathic nephrotic syndrome should be closely monitored for the development of malignancy during the year following diagnosis. Because both the renal histology and prognosis of patients with malignancy-related nephrotic syndrome generally parallel the underlying disease, our policy has been to withhold renal biopsy except for patients in whom heavy proteinuria persists despite remission of the neoplasm.

Although heavy proteinuria is a common feature of multiple myeloma, the nephrotic syndrome is a relatively rare complication of myeloma or other paraproteinemias. In more than 90% of patients with multiple myeloma, proteinuria results chiefly from increased light chain excretion. Marked albuminuria, sufficient to result in the frank nephrotic syndrome, generally results from amyloidosis or light chain nephropathy.[117, 118] Light chain nephropathy is a unique glomerulopathy resulting from the deposition of light chains within the mesangium and GBM.[119] While over one third of patients have coexistent myeloma, the majority demonstrate only increased urinary light chain excretion, often in conjunction with a monoclonal serum light chain. Most cases of light chain nephropathy occur in men in the fifth to seventh decade. Renal insufficiency is frequent at the time of diagnosis, nonselective proteinuria common, and the nephrotic syndrome present in approximately 30%.[119] Renal biopsy demonstrates nodular mesangial deposition of eosinophilic material resembling amyloidosis or diabetic glomerulosclerosis. Immunofluorescent staining is negative for classical immunoglobulins and complement, but positive with specific antisera to kappa or lambda light chains. Electron microscopic examination reveals continuous subendothelial electron-dense material and granular electron-dense mesangial deposits. There is no specific therapy for light chain nephropathy. Treatment directed at associated myeloma rarely influences the renal manifestations. Approximately one third progress to ESRD and require long-term dialytic support.[119] Heavy nonselective proteinuria has been described occasionally in Waldenstrom's macroglobulinemia and in benign monoclonal gammopathies,[120, 121] however these paraproteinemias are uncommon causes of the nephrotic syndrome.

INFECTIOUS DISEASES

Because many glomerulopathies are immunologically mediated, it is not surprising that a variety of infectious processes are associated with heavy proteinuria (Table 4–1). Fortunately, effective antimicrobial therapy is available for many and usually results in gradual resolution of the renal manifestations. It is important to consider a number of infectious etiologies in any patient with otherwise unexplained nephrotic range proteinuria.

Poststreptococcal Glomerulonephritis

Poststreptococcal glomerulonephritis is primarily a disease of children between the ages of 3 and 8 years. With increasing age the prevalence of streptococcal disease and its sequelae decline. However, attack rates are variable and large series of adults with acute poststreptococcal glomerulonephritis (APSGN) have been described.[122–124] In contrast to rheumatic fever, only certain nephritogenic types of streptococci are associated with APSGN. Ten serotypes (types 1, 2, 3, 4, 12, 25, 49, 55, 57, 60), based on the specific M protein of the streptococcal cell wall, are most frequently implicated in APSGN.[122] Although APSGN may occur with an incidence as high as 20% after streptococcal pharyngitis or pyoderma, overt renal manifestations are uncommon and the nephrotic syndrome unusual.

The clinical manifestations of APSGN occur after a latent period of one to two weeks and characteristically consist of hematuria, proteinuria, edema, and hypertension. A positive streptozyme test, which detects antibodies to five different streptococcal antigens, occurs in over 90% of cases; serum complement levels are decreased during the first two weeks of illness in over 95%.[122] Urinary protein excretion is usually less than 2 gm per 24 hours, particularly in children. Some series with a predominance of adult patients, however, have reported the nephrotic syndrome in 20% of clinically apparent cases.[123] Such series are unusual and undoubtedly overestimate the frequency of the nephrotic syndrome in APSGN.

Renal histologic findings are characteristic in APSGN if the biopsy is obtained during the first three to six weeks of the illness. The glomeruli are hypercellular due to both endothelial and mesangial cell proliferation (Fig 4–10,A). Immunofluorescence microscopy discloses a coarse granular deposition of C3 and IgG along the capillary loops and within the mesangium. Characteristic, large, subepithelial, electron-dense deposits are seen with electron microscopy (Fig 4–10,B),

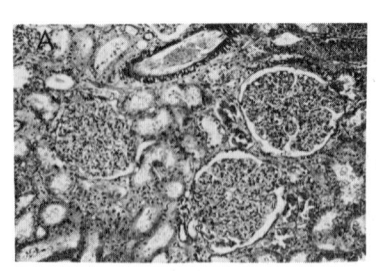

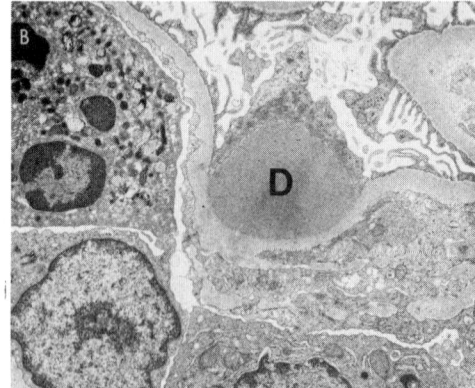

Fig 4–10.—Renal biopsy material from a patient with acute poststreptococcal glomerulonephritis. **A,** hematoxylin- and eosin-stained section showing enlarged, hypercellular glomeruli. **B,** electron micrograph of a capillary loop demonstrating a characteristic large subepithelial electron dense deposit *(D)*.

as are occasional smaller, mesangial, intramembranous and subendothelial deposits. The pathologic findings in APSGN suggest that the glomerular lesion results from deposition of immune-complexes; however, circulating immune-complexes of streptococcal antigen and antibody have been difficult to detect.[122] The possibility that streptococcal antigens are deposited within the GBM and elicit in situ immune-complex formation is an attractive hypothesis but has been difficult to confirm.

There is no specific treatment for APSGN. Therapy should be directed at control of blood pressure and edema formation. Long-term studies of both epidemic and endemic APSGN have demonstrated clinical resolution in over 95% of cases[125]; however, Baldwin and coworkers have suggested that the prognosis may be poorer in adults with endemic APSGN. In their studies, the nephrotic syndrome occurred in 20% of patients early in the course of APSGN but resolved in the majority. The persistence of heavy proteinuria in a small number of patients was associated with progressive glomerulosclerosis and the development of ESRD.[123, 124]

Bacterial Endocarditis

Clinically apparent renal involvement occurs frequently in bacterial endocarditis and histologic evidence of glomerulonephritis is present in virtually all cases.[126, 127] During the past two decades, the clinical spectrum of endocarditis has shifted due to a decrease in the prevalence of rheumatic heart disease, the widespread availability of antibiotics, and an increase in the incidence of drug abuse. Acute endocarditis due to *Staphylococcus aureus* has replaced subacute endocarditis due to *Streptococcus viridans* as the leading cause of bacterial endocarditis. In spite of the changing epidemiology, glomerulonephritis remains a common feature of bacterial endocarditis and is clinically evident in 40% to 80% of reported cases. Neugarten and Baldwin recently reviewed the literature and found that the nephrotic syndrome was present in 14% (20 of 126) of cases with histologically documented glomerulonephritis.[126]

The glomerulonephritis of bacterial endocarditis is probably an immune-complex disease. In most patients with endocarditis, hypocomplementemia and circulating immune-complexes are readily demonstrable.[128] Furthermore, bacterial antigens and specific antibody directed against the causative organism have been identified in glomerular tissue.[126, 129] It has not been determined whether the circulating complexes deposit within the glomerulus or whether antigen is fixed within the GBM resulting in in situ complex formation. By light microscopy the histologic changes range from a focal segmental to diffuse proliferative glomerulonephritis (DPGN). Immunofluorescent staining reveals C3, IgG, IgM, and IgA in various combinations in both the mesangium and GBM. Acute endocarditis with *S. aureus* is usually associated with large subepithelial electron dense deposits very similar to those found in APSGN. Subacute endocarditis due to less virulent organisms generally results in mesangial and subendothelial deposits.[126, 128]

There is no specific treatment for the glomerulonephritis or nephrotic syndrome of bacterial endocarditis. With adequate antimicrobial therapy and resolution of the endocarditis, the renal manifestations gradually subside. *S. aureus* endocarditis is usually associated with DPGN, an increased frequency of the nephrotic syndrome, and occasionally with the development of acute renal failure. Despite these ominous signs, the vast majority of patients recover normal renal function with appropriate treatment. Rarely, dialysis is required until adequate renal function returns. Non-staphylococcal endocarditis is usually associated with a less severe histologic picture, lesser frequency of heavy proteinuria, and generally well-preserved renal function. Under the latter circumstances, microscopic hematuria and proteinuria usually resolve within several weeks of effective antibiotic treatment.[126]

Hepatitis B

Glomerulonephritis, often associated with the nephrotic syndrome, is an important extrahepatic manifestation of chronic hepatitis B antigenemia. A variety of renal lesions have been associated with hepatitis B infection including membranous, membranoproliferative, and mesangioproliferative glomerulopathies.[130, 131] The pathogenesis of the glomerulonephritis associated with hepatitis B appears to involve either the deposition of circulating immune-complexes of viral antigen and antibody within the glomerulus, or to in situ complex formation after viral antigens become fixed within the GBM. The major hepatitis B antigens, HB_sAg, HB_cAg and HB_eAg, have all been identified in the glomeruli of patients with chronic HB_sAg antigenemia and proteinuria.[130-134] Recent studies suggest that HB_eAg may be most frequently linked to the development of membranous glomerulopathy.[134] The natural history of the glomerulopathies due to hepatitis B is unknown. Numerous studies have described histopathology and explored the pathogenesis, but no long-term study has adequately described the clinical course of a large number of patients.

Other Infectious Diseases

Well-documented cases of the nephrotic syndrome have occurred in conjunction with secondary syphilis, malaria, schistosomiasis, and viral infections. However, these causes of the secondary nephrotic syndrome are usually easily recognized and represent clinical curiosities rather than frequent associations.

PREGNANCY

The nephrotic syndrome complicates pregnancy with a frequency of approximately one to two cases per 1000 deliveries.[135, 136] The exact cause of heavy proteinuria during pregnancy has been difficult to estimate because most nephrologists are reluctant to recommend renal biopsy in pregnant patients. Nevertheless, the results of several carefully conducted studies have provided valuable information regarding the etiology, effect on maternal and fetal morbidity, and natural history of pregnancy-associated nephrotic syndrome.

Normal pregnancy is associated with increments in cardiac output, renal blood flow and GFR, and altered tubular handling of glucose and amino acids; however, there is no appreciable change in tubular reabsorption of protein.[135] Thus, the finding of proteinuria in pregnancy strongly suggests the presence of underlying renal disease; heavy proteinuria implies significant glomerular pathology.

The frequency and types of renal lesions associated with the nephrotic syndrome in pregnancy vary with the patient population and selection criteria. Fisher and co-workers found that 27 of 100 patients with hypertensive pregnancies had proteinuria greater than 3.5 gm/24 hours.[136] Glomerular capillary endotheliosis, a pathologic hallmark of preeclampsia characterized by diffuse swelling of endothelial cells and deposits of fibrin-like material between the endothelial cell and GBM, was the only renal lesion in 23 of 27 subjects. An additional six normotensive nephrotic patients did not undergo renal biopsy. Thus, in this series, preeclampsia accounted for at least two thirds of all cases of the nephrotic syndrome during pregnancy, and the authors concluded that preeclampsia was the most common cause of pregnancy-associated nephrotic syndrome.[136] By contrast, European investigators have found glomerular capillary endotheliosis in less than one half of patients with clinically diagnosed preeclampsia; the majority exhibited a variety of primary glomerulopathies.[137, 138] The distribution of glomerular lesions roughly paralleled that of an age-matched population. Membranoproliferative glomerulonephritis, focal glomerulosclerosis, and IgA nephropathy each accounted for 15% of biopsy-proven glomerular disease, while mesangioproliferative glomerulonephritis, membranous glomerulopathy, and minimal change disease occurred with a lesser frequency.[137, 138]

The clinical course of patients who develop the nephrotic syndrome during pregnancy depends on the underlying histopathology, the presence or absence of coexistent hypertension, and GFR. In general, patients with biopsy-proven preeclampsia, normal renal function and mild hypertension have a good prognosis despite heavy proteinuria.[136] Long-term follow-up in these subjects has shown persistence of normal renal function and resolution of proteinuria in all cases. The clinical course is more variable in patients with primary glomerular disease.[139] Patients with mild hypertension and minimal renal insufficiency exhibit only a slight increase in maternal and fetal complications. However, severe hypertension and moderate renal insufficiency are associated with an incidence of fetal wastage as high as 15%.[135, 138, 139] Most workers agree that pregnancy per se does not adversely affect the rate of progression of underlying renal disease.[140]

Based on the above considerations, we avoid renal biopsy in pregnant patients unless antithrombotic therapy is contemplated in a patient with rapidly deteriorating renal function. Primiparous patients with no history of renal disease and only mild hypertension are likely to have true preeclampsia with a good long-term prognosis. Subjects with documented preexisting proteinuria or multiparous patients who develop the nephrotic syndrome generally have a preexisting renal lesion that has become clinically more apparent with pregnancy. Under these circumstances, the nephrotic syndrome usually resolves postpartum; if heavy proteinuria persists following delivery, however, renal biopsy should be considered as in other patients with nephrotic syndrome.

MISCELLANEOUS CAUSES OF NEPHROTIC SYNDROME

In addition to the previously described causes of secondary nephrotic syndrome, heavy proteinuria has been well documented with varying frequency in patients with glomerular disease due to Wegener's granulomatosis,[141–143] sickle cell anemia,[84, 144] essential mixed cryoglobulinema,[145, 146] Henoch-Schönlein purpura,[147] polyarteritis nodosa,[148] Alport's syndrome,[149, 150] chronic allograft rejection,[151] vesicoureteral reflux,[152, 153] and renal artery stenosis.[154] The renal histopathology in these disorders frequently consists of a nonspecific focal or diffuse proliferative glomerulonephritis but, in some cases, resembles lesions primarily associated with the idiopathic nephrotic syndrome (Table 6–2). In most instances, identification of the primary disease predicts the renal histology, and biopsy is not required. Effective treatment of the underlying disorder often results in resolution of the nephrotic syndrome.

REFERENCES

1. Mitchell J.C.: End-stage renal failure in juvenile diabetes mellitus. *Mayo Clin. Proc.* 52:281, 1977.
2. Goldstein D.A., Massry S.G.: Diabetic nephropathy: clinical course and effect of hemodialysis. *Nephron* 20:286, 1978.
3. Fabre J., Balant L.P., Dayer P.G., et al.: The kidney in maturity onset diabetes mellitus: A clinical study of 510 patients. *Kidney Int.* 21:730, 1982.
4. Goetz F.C., Kjellstrand C.M.: The treatment of diabetic kidney disease. *Diabetologia* 17:267, 1979.
5. Friedman E.A.: Diabetic nephropathy: strategies in prevention and management. *Kidney Int.* 21:780, 1982.
6. Rettig B., Teutsch S.M.: The incidence of end-stage renal disease in type I and type II diabetes mellitus. *Diabetic Nephropathy* 3:26, 1984.
7. Mauer S.M., Barbosa J., Vernier R.L., et al.: Development of diabetic vascular lesions in normal kidneys transplanted into patients with diabetes mellitus. *N. Engl. J. Med.* 295:916, 1976.
8. Mogensen C.E.: Renal function changes in diabetes. *Diabetes* 25:872, 1976.
9. Herf S., Pohl S.L., Sturgill B., et al.: An evaluation of diabetic and pseudodiabetic glomerulosclerosis. *Am. J. Med.* 66:1040, 1979.
10. Wahl P., Depperman D., Hasslacher C.: Biochemistry of glomerular basement membrane of the normal and diabetic human. *Kidney Int.* 21:744, 1982.
11. Friedman E.A.: Clinical imperatives in diabetic nephropathy. *Kidney Int.* 23:S-16, 1983.
12. Mogensen C.E., Osterby R., Gundersen H.J.G.: Early functional and morphologic vascular renal consequences of the diabetic state. *Diabetologica* 17:71, 1979.
13. Hostetter T.H., Rennke H.G., Brenner B.M.: The case for intrarenal hypertension in the initiation and progression of diabetic and other glomerulopathies. *Am. J. Med.* 72:375, 1982.
14. Viberti G.C., Pickup J.C., Jarrett R.J., et al.: Effect of control of blood glucose on urinary excretion of albumin and B_2 microglobulin in insulin-dependent diabetes. *N. Engl. J. Med.* 300:638, 1979.
15. Viberti G.C., Wiseman M.J.: The natural history of proteinuria in insulin-dependent diabetes mellitus. *Diabetic Nephropathy* 2:22, 1983.
16. Mogensen C.E.: Microalbuminuria predicts clinical proteinuria and early mortality in maturity-onset diabetes. *N. Engl. J. Med.* 310:356, 1984.
17. Carrie B.J., Myers B.D.: Proteinuria and functional characteristics of the glomerular barrier in diabetic nephropathy. *Kidney Int.* 17:669, 1980.

18. Myers B.D., Winetz J.A., Chui F., et al.: Mechanisms of proteinuria in diabetic nephropathy: A study of glomerular barrier function. *Kidney Int.* 17:669, 1980.
19. Meyer T.W., Anderson S., Brenner B.M.: Dietary protein intake and progressive glomerular sclerosis: The role of capillary hypertension and hyperperfusion in the progression of renal disease. *Ann. Intern. Med.* 98:832, 1983.
20. Mogensen C.E.: Diabetes mellitus and the kidney. *Kidney Int.* 21:673, 1982.
21. Mogensen C.E., Christensen C.K.: Predicting diabetic nephropathy in insulin dependent patients. *N. Engl. J. Med.* 311:89, 1984.
22. Kussman M.J., Goldstein A., Gleason R.E.: The clinical course of diabetic nephropathy. *J.A.M.A.* 236:1861, 1976.
23. Viberti G.C., Bilous R.W., Mackintosh D., et al.: Monitoring glomerular function in diabetic nephropathy: A prospective study. *Am. J. Med.* 74:256, 1983.
24. Chaha P.S., Kohner E.M.: The relationship between diabetic retinopathy and diabetic nephropathy. *Diabetic Nephropathy* 2:4, 1983.
25. Mogensen C.E.: Hypertension in diabetes and the stages of diabetic nephropathy. *Diabetic Nephropathy* 1:2, 1982.
26. O'Neill W.M., Wallin J.D. Walker P.D.: Hematuria and red cell casts in typical diabetic nephropathy. *Am. J. Med.* 74:389, 1983.
27. Rao K.V., Crosson J.T.: Idiopathic membranous glomerulonephritis in diabetic patients. *Arch. Intern. Med.* 140:624, 1980.
28. Kasinath B.S., Mujars S.K., Spargo B.H., et al.: Nondiabetic renal disease in patients with diabetes mellitus. *Am. J. Med.* 75:613, 1983.
29. Carstens S.A., Herbert L.A., Garancis J.C., et al.: Rapidly progressive glomerulonephritis superimposed on diabetic glomerulosclerosis. *J.A.M.A.* 247:1453, 1982.
30. Deckert T., Laritzen T., Parving H.H., et al.: Effect of two years of strict metabolic control on kidney function in long-term insulin-dependent diabetics. *Diabetic Nephropathy* 2:6, 1983.
31. Cataland S., O'Dorisio T.M.: Diabetic nephropathy: Clinical course in patients treated with the subcutaneous insulin pump. *J.A.M.A.* 249:2059, 1983.
32. Mogensen C.E.: Long-term antihypertensive treatment inhibiting progression of diabetic nephropathy. *Br. Med. J.* 285:685, 1982.
33. Vollmer W.M., Wahl P.W., Blagg C.R.: Survival with dialysis and transplantation in patients with end-stage renal disease. *N. Engl. J. Med.* 308:1553, 1983.
34. Richmond J.D., Sturgill B.C., Bolton W.K.: Recurrence of typical diffuse and nodular diabetic glomerulosclerosis in a renal allograft of a diabetic patient: Functional deterioration in a six year old graft. *Diabetic Nephropathy* 3:28, 1984.
35. Cameron J.S., Turner D.R., Ogg C.S., et al.: Systemic lupus with nephritis. A long-term study. *Q.J. Med.* 48:1, 1979.
36. Decker J.L., Steinberg A.D., Reinesteen J.L., et al.: Systemic lupus erythmatosus: Evolving concepts. *Ann. Intern. Med.* 91:587, 1979.
37. Mahajan S.K., Ordonez N.G., Feitelson P.J., et al.: Lupus nephropathy without clinical renal involvement. *Medicine* 56:493, 1977.
38. Austin H.A., Muenz L.R., Joyce K.M., et al.: Prognostic factors in lupus nephritis: Contribution of renal histologic data. *Am. J. Med.* 75:382, 1983.
39. Baldwin D.S., Gluck M.C., Lowenstein J., et al.: Lupus nephritis: Clinical course as related to morphologic forms and their transitions. *Am. J. Med.* 62:12, 1977.
40. Austin H.A., Meunz L.R., Joyce K.M., et al.: Diffuse proliferative lupus nephritis: Identification of specific pathologic features affecting renal outcome. *Kidney Int.* 25:689, 1984.
41. Jennette J.C., Iskandai S.S., Dalldorf F.G.: Pathologic differentiation between lupus and nonlupus membranous glomerulopathy. *Kidney Int.* 24:377, 1983.
42. Lewis E.J., Busch G.J., Schur P.H.: Gamma G globulin subgroup composition of the glomerular deposits in human renal diseases. *J. Clin. Invest.* 49:1103, 1970.
43. Gershwin M.E., Steinberg A.D.: Qualitative characteristics of anti-DNA antibodies in lupus nephritis. *Arthritis Rheum.* 17:947, 1974.

44. Pennebaker J., Gilliam J.N., Ziff M.: Significance of anti-nDNA classes in serum and skin in prognosis of SLE. *Arthritis Rheum.* 19:815, 1976.
45. Koffler D., Agnello V., Kunkel H.G.: Polynucleotide immune complexes in serum and glomeruli of patients with systemic lupus erythematosus. *Am. J. Pathol.* 74:109, 1974.
46. Eiser A.R., Katz S.M., Swartz C.: Clinically occult diffuse proliferative lupus nephritis. *Arch. Intern. Med.* 139:1022, 1979.
47. Fries J.F., Porta J., Liang M.H.: Marginal benefit of renal biopsy in systemic lupus erythematosus. *Arch. Intern. Med.* 138:1386, 1978.
48. Carette S., Klippel J.H., Decker J.L., et al.: Controlled studies of oral immunosuppressive drugs in lupus nephritis. *Ann. Intern. Med.* 99:1, 1983.
49. Jarrett M.P., Santhanam S., DelGreco F.: The clinical course of end-stage renal disease in systemic lupus erythematosus. *Arch. Intern. Med.* 143:1353, 1983.
50. Cheigh J.S., Stenzel K.H., Rubin A.L., et al.: Systemic lupus erythematosus in patients with chronic renal failure. *Am. J. Med.* 75:602, 1983.
51. Coplon N.S., Diskin C.J., Petersen J., et al.: The long-term clinical course of systemic lupus erythematosus in end-stage renal disease. *N. Engl. J. Med.* 308:186, 1983.
52. Kimberly R.P., Lockshin M.D., Sherman R.L., et al.: Reversible "end-stage" lupus nephritis: Analysis of patients able to discontinue dialysis. *Am. J. Med.* 74:361, 1983.
53. Jarrett M.P., Sablay L.B., Walter L., et al.: The effect of continuous normalization of serum hemolytic complement on the course of lupus nephritis. *Am. J. Med.* 70:1067, 1981.
54. Kimberly R.P., Lockshin M.D., Sherman R.L., et al.: High-dose intravenous methylprednisolone pulse therapy in systemic lupus erythematosus. *Am. J. Med.* 70:817, 1981.
55. Balow J.E., Austin H.A., Muenz L.R., et al.: Effect of treatment on the evolution of renal abnormalities in lupus nephritis. *N. Engl. J. Med.* 311:491, 1984.
56. Plotz P.H., Klippel J.H., Decker J.L., et al.: Bladder complications in patients receiving cyclophosphamide for systemic lupus erythematosus or rheumatoid arthritis. *Ann. Intern. Med.* 91:221, 1979.
57. Elliott R.W., Essenhigh D.M., Morley A.R.: Cyclophosphamide treatment of systemic lupus erythematosus: Risk of bladder cancer exceeds benefit. *Br. Med. J.* 284:1160, 1982.
58. Steinberg A.F.: Cyclophosphamide. Should it be used daily, monthly or never. *N. Engl. J. Med.* 310:458, 1984.
59. Dinant H.J., Decker J.L., Klippel J.H.: Alternative modes of cyclophosphamide and azathioprine therapy in lupus nephritis. *Ann. Intern. Med.* 96:728, 1982.
60. Donadio J.V.: Cytotoxic-drug treatment of lupus nephritis. *N. Engl. J. Med.* 311:528, 1984.
61. Amend W.J.C., Vincenti F., Feduska N.J., et al.: Recurrent systemic lupus erythematosus involving renal allografts. *N. Engl. J. Med.* 94:444, 1981.
62. Cornwell G.G., Murdock W.L., Kyle R.A., et al.: Frequency and distribution of senile cardiovascular amyloid: a clinicopathologic correlation. *Am. J. Med.* 75:618, 1983.
63. Glenner G.G.: Amyloid deposits and amyloidosis. *N. Engl. J. Med.* 302:1283, 1333, 1980.
64. Franklin E.C.: Some unsolved problems in the amyloid diseases. *Am. J. Med.* 66:365, 1979.
65. Durie B.G.M., Persky B., Soehnlen B.J., et al.: Amyloid production in human myeloma stem-cell culture, with morphologic evidence of amyloid secretion by associated macrophages. *N. Engl. J. Med.* 307:1689, 1982.
66. Scholes J., Derasena R., Appel G.B., et al.: Amyloidosis in chronic heroin addicts with the nephrotic syndrome. *Ann. Intern. Med.* 91:26, 1979.

67. Pras M., Zaretzky J., Frangione B., et al.: AA protein in a case of "primary" or "idiopathic" amyloidosis. *Am. J. Med.* 68:291, 1980.
68. Huston D.P., McAdam K.P., Balow J.E., et al.: Amyloidosis in systemic lupus erythematosus. *Am. J. Med.* 70:320, 1981.
69. Pras M., Franklin E.C., Shibolet S., et al.: Amyloidosis associated with renal cell carcinoma of the AA type. *Am. J. Med.* 73:426, 1982.
70. Kyle R.A., Bayrd E.O.: Amyloidosis: review of 236 cases. *Medicine* 54:271, 1975.
71. Ben Ari J., Zlotnick M., Oren A., et al.: Dialysis in renal failure caused by amyloidosis of familial Mediterranean fever. *Arch. Intern. Med.* 136:449, 1976.
72. Cohen H.J., Lessin L.S., Hallal J., et al.: Resolution of primary amyloidosis during chemotherapy. *Ann. Intern. Med.* 82:466, 1975.
73. Boxbaum J.N., Hurley M.E., Chuba J., et al.: Amyloidosis of the AL type: Clinical, morphologic and biochemical aspects of the response to therapy with alkylating agents and prednisone. *Am. J. Med.* 67:867, 1979.
74. Ravid M., Robson M., Kedar I.: Prolonged colchicine treatment in four patients with amyloidosis. *Ann. Intern. Med.* 87:568, 1977.
75. Ravid M., Shapiro J., Lang R., et al.: Prolonged dimethylsulphoxide treatment in 13 patients with systemic amyloidosis. *Ann. Rheum. Dis.* 41:587, 1982.
76. Light P.D., Hall-Craggs M.: Amyloid deposition in a renal allograft in a case of amyloidosis secondary to rheumatoid arthritis. *Am. J. Med.* 66:532, 1979.
77. Bennett W.M., Plamp C., Porter G.A.: Drug related syndromes in clinical nephrology. *Ann. Intern. Med.* 87:582, 1977.
78. Roxe D.M.: Toxic nephropathy from diagnostic and therapeutic agents. *Am. J. Med.* 69:759, 1980.
79. Vaamonde C.A., Hunt F.R.: The nephrotic syndrome as a complication of gold therapy. *Arthritis Rheum.* 13:826, 1970.
80. Tornroth T., Skrifvars B.: Gold nephropathy prototype of membranous glomerulonephritis. *Am. J. Pathol.* 75:573, 1974.
81. Samuels B., Lee J.C., Engleman E.P., et al.: Membranous nephropathy in patients with rheumatoid arthritis: relationship to gold therapy. *Medicine* 57:319, 1977.
82. Plaza J.J., Herrero G., Barat A., et al.: Membranous glomerulonephritis as a complication of oral gold therapy. *Ann. Intern. Med.* 97:563, 1982.
83. Katz W.A., Blodgett R.C., Pietrusko R.G.: Proteinuria in gold-treated rheumatoid arthritis. *Ann. Intern. Med.* 101:176, 1984.
84. Pardo V., Strauss J., Kramer H., et al.: Nephropathy associated with sickle cell anemia: An autologous immune complex nephritis: II. Clinicopathologic study of seven patients. *Am. J. Med.* 59:650, 1975.
85. Douglas M.F.S., Rabideau D.P., Schwartz M.M., et al.: Evidence of autologous immune-complex nephritis. *N. Engl. J. Med.* 305:1326, 1981.
86. Brezin J.H., Katz S.M., Schwartz A.B., et al.: Reversible renal failure and nephrotic syndrome associated with nonsteroidal anti-inflammatory drugs. *N. Engl. J. Med.* 301:1271, 1979.
87. Curt G.A., Kaldany A., Whitley L.G., et al.: Reversible rapidly progressive renal failure with nephrotic syndrome due to fenoprofen calcium. *Ann. Intern. Med.* 92:72, 1980.
88. Finkelstein A., Fraley D.S., Stachura I., et al.: Fenoprofen nephropathy: Lipoid nephrosis and interstitial nephritis. *Am. J. Med.* 72:81, 1982.
89. Stachura I., Jayakumar S., Bourke E.: T and B lymphocyte subsets in fenoprofen nephropathy. *Am. J. Med.* 75:9, 1983.
90. Clive D.M., Stoff J.S.: Renal syndromes associated with nonsteroidal anti-inflammatory drugs. *N. Engl. J. Med.* 310:563, 1984.
91. Bender W.L., Whelton A., Beschorner W.E., et al.: Interstitial nephritis, proteinuria, and renal failure caused by nonsteroidal anti-inflammatory drugs. *Am. J. Med.* 76:1006, 1984.
92. Vidt D.G., Bravo E.L., Fouad F.M.: Captopril. *N. Engl. J. Med.* 306:214, 1982.

93. Textor S.C., Gephardt G.N., Bravo E.L., et al.: Membranous glomerulopathy associated with captopril therapy. *Am. J. Med.* 74:705, 1983.
94. Hoorntje S.J., Weening J.J., The T.H., et al.: Immune-complex glomerulopathy in patients treated with captopril. *Lancet* 1:1212, 1980.
95. Hoorntje S.J., Donker A.J.M., Prins E.J.L., et al.: Membranous glomerulopathy in a patient on captopril. *Acta Med. Scand.* 208:325, 1980.
96. Meador K.H., Sharon Z., Lewis E.J.: Renal amyloidosis and subcutaneous drug abuse. *Ann. Intern. Med.* 91:565, 1979.
97. Rao T.K.S., Nicastri A.D., Friedman E.A.: Natural history of heroin-associated nephropathy. *N. Engl. J. Med.* 290:19, 1974.
98. Treser G., Cherubin C., Lonergan E.T., et al.: Renal lesions in narcotic addicts. *Am. J. Med.* 57:687, 1974.
99. Cunningham E.E., Brentjens J.R., Zielezny M.A., et al.: Heroin nephropathy: a clinicopathologic and epidemiologic study. *Am. J. Med.* 68:47, 1980.
100. Cunningham E.E., Zielezny M.A., Venuto R.C.: Heroin-associated nephropathy. *J.A.M.A.* 250:2935, 1983.
101. Bacon P.A., Tribe C.R., Mackenzie J.L., et al.: Penicillamine nephropathy in rheumatoid arthritis. *Q. J. Med.* 45:661, 1976.
102. Stein H.B., Patterson A.C., Offer R.C., et al.: Adverse effects of D-Penicillamine in rheumatoid arthritis. *Ann. Intern. Med.* 92:24, 1980.
103. Richman A.V., Masco H.L., Rifkin S.I., et al.: Minimal change disease and the nephrotic syndrome associated with lithium therapy. *Ann. Intern. Med.* 92:70, 1980.
104. Watson A.J.S., Dalbow M.H., Stachura I., et al.: Immunologic studies in cimetidine-induced nephropathy and polymyositis. *N. Engl. J. Med.* 308:142, 1983.
105. Appel G.B., D'Agati V., Bergman M., et al.: Nephrotic syndrome and immune complex glomerulonephritis associated with chlorpropamide therapy. *Am. J. Med.* 74:337, 1983.
106. Gagliano R.G., Costanzi J.J., Beathard G.A., et al.: The nephrotic syndrome associated with neoplasia: An unusual paraneoplastic syndrome. *Am. J. Med.* 60:1026, 1976.
107. Eagan J.W., Lewis E.J.: Glomerulopathies of neoplasia. *Kidney Int.* 11:297–306, 1977.
108. Fer M.F., McKinney T.D., Richardson R.L., et al.: Cancer and the kidney: Renal complications of neoplasms. *Am. J. Med.* 71:704, 1981.
109. Row P.G., Cameron J.S., Turner D.R., et al.: Membranous nephropathy. Long-term follow-up in association with neoplasia. *Q. J. Med.* 44:207, 1975.
110. Zimmerman S.W., Moorthy A.V., Burkholder P.M., et al.: Glomerulopathies associated with neoplastic disease, in Rieselbach R.E., Garnick M.B. (eds.): *Cancer and the Kidney*. Philadelphia, Lea & Febiger, 1982, pp. 306–378.
111. Moorthy A.V., Zimmerman S.W., Burkholder P.M.: Nephrotic syndrome in Hodgkin's disease: Evidence for a pathogenesis alternative to immune complex deposition. *Am. J. Med.* 61:471, 1976.
112. Couser W.G., Wagonfeld J.B., Spargo B.H., et al.: Glomerular deposition of tumor antigen in membranous nephropathy associated with colonic carcinoma. *Am. J. Med.* 57:962, 1974.
113. Ozawa T., Pluss R., Lacher J., et al.: Endogenous immune complex nephropathy associated with malignancy: I. Studies on the nature and immunopathogenetic significance of glomerular bound antigen and antibody, isolation and characterization of tumor specific antigen and antibody and circulating immune complexes. *Q. J. Med.* 44:523, 1975.
114. Costanza M.E., Pinn V., Schwartz R.S., et al.: Carcinoembryonic antigen-antibody complexes in a patient with colonic carcinoma and nephrotic syndrome. *N. Engl. J. Med.* 289:520, 1973.
115. Couser W., Badger A., Cooperband S., et al.: Hodgkin's disease and lipoid nephrosis. *Lancet* 1:912, 1977.

116. Barton C.H., Vaziri N.D., Spear G.S.: Nephrotic syndrome associated with adenocarcinoma of the breast. *Am. J. Med.* 68:308, 1980.
117. Martinez-Maldonado M., Yium J., Suki W.N., et al.: Renal complications in multiple myeloma: Pathophysiology and some aspects of clinical management. *J. Chronic Dis.* 24:221, 1971.
118. DeFronzo R.A., Cooke C.R., Wright J.R., et al.: Renal function in patients with multiple myeloma. *Medicine* 57:151, 1978.
119. Tubbs R.R., Gephardt G.N., McMachon J.T., et al.: Light chain nephropathy. *Am. J. Med.* 71:263, 1981.
120. Zlotnick A., Rosenmann E.: Renal pathologic findings associated with monoclonal gammopathies. *Arch. Intern. Med.* 35:40, 1975.
121. Avasthi P.S., Erickson D.G., Williams R.C., et al.: Benign monoclonal gammaglobulinemia and glomerulonephritis. *Am. J. Med.* 62:324, 1977.
122. Nissenson A.R., Baroff L.J., Fine R.N., et al.: Poststreptococcal acute glomerulonephritis: fact and controversy. *Ann. Intern. Med.* 91:76, 1979.
123. Baldwin D.S., Gluck M.C., Schacht R.G., et al.: The long-term course of poststreptococcal glomerulonephritis. *Ann. Intern Med.* 80:342, 1974.
124. Schacht R.G., Gluck M.C., Gallo G.R., et al.: Progression to uremia after remission of acute poststreptococcal glomerulonephritis. *N. Engl. J. Med.* 295:977, 1976.
125. Potter E.V., Lipschitz S.A., Abidh S., et al.: Twelve to seventeen-year follow-up of patients with poststreptococcal acute glomerulonephritis in Trinidad. *N. Engl. J. Med.* 307:725, 1982.
126. Neugarten J., Baldwin D.S.: Glomerulonephritis in bacterial endocarditis. *Am. J. Med.* 77:297, 1984.
127. Morel-Maroger L., Sraer J.D., Herreman G., et al.: Kidney in subacute endocarditis. *Arch. Pathol. Lab. Med.* 94:205, 1972.
128. Gutman R.A., Striker G.E., Gilliland B.C., et al.: The immune complex glomerulonephritis of bacterial endocarditis. *Medicine* 51:1, 1972.
129. Levy R.L., Hong R.: The immune nature of subacute bacterial endocarditis nephritis. *Am. J. Med.* 54:645, 1973.
130. Brzosko W.J., Krawczynski K., Nazorewicz T., et al.: Glomerulonephritis associated with hepatitis-B surface antigen immune complexes in children. *Lancet* 2:477, 1974.
131. Nagy J., Bajtai G., Brasch H., et al.: The role of hepatitis B surface antigen in the pathogenesis of glomerulopathies. *Clin. Nephrol.* 12:109, 1979.
132. Kohler P.F., Cronin R.E., Hammond W.S., et al.: Chronic membranous glomerulonephritis caused by hepatitis B antigen-antibody immune complexes. *Ann. Intern. Med.* 81:448, 1974.
133. Takekoshi Y., Tanaka M., Miyakawa Y., et al.: Free "small" and IgG-associated "large" hepatitis B_e antigen in the serum and glomerular capillary walls of two patients with membranous glomerulonephritis. *N. Engl. J. Med.* 300:814, 1979.
134. Hirose H., Udo K., Kojima M., et al.: Deposition of hepatitis B_e antigen in membranous glomerulonephritis: identification by $F(ab')_2$ fragments of monoclonal antibody. *Kidney Int.* 26:338, 1984.
135. Zacur H.A., Mitch W.E.: Renal disease in pregnancy. *Med. Clin. North Am.* 61:89, 1977.
136. Fisher K.A., Ahuja S., Luger A., et al.: Nephrotic proteinuria with pre-eclampsia. *Am. J. Obstet. Gynecol.* 129:643, 1977.
137. Beller F.K., Dame W.R., Witting Ch.: Renal disease diagnosed by renal biopsy. *Contrib. Nephrol.* 25:61, 1981.
138. Surian M., Imbasciatti E., Cosci P., et al: Glomerular disease and pregnancy. *Nephron* 36:101, 1984.
139. Ferris T.F.: The kidney in pregnancy, in Earley L.E., Gottschalk, C.W. (eds.): *Strauss and Welt's Diseases of the Kidney.* Boston, Little, Brown & Co., 1979, pp. 1321–1356.

140. Katz A.I., Lindheimer M.D.: Effect of pregnancy on the natural course of kidney disease. *Seminars in Nephrol.* 4:252, 1984.
141. Horn R.G., Fauci A.S., Rosenthal A.S., et al.: Renal biopsy pathology in Wegener's granulomatosis. *Am. J. Pathol.* 74:423, 1974.
142. Wolff S.M., Fauci A.S., Horn R.G., et al.: Wegener's granulomatosis. *Ann. Intern. Med.* 81:513, 1974.
143. Fauci A.S., Haynes B.F., Katz P., et al.: Wegener's granulomatosis: prospective clinical and therapeutic experience with 85 patients for 21 years. *Ann. Intern. Med.* 98:76, 1983.
144. Alleyne G.A.O., Statius Van Eps L.W., Addae S.K., et al.: The kidney in sickle cell anemia. *Kidney Int.* 7:371, 1975.
145. Gorevic P.D., Kassab H.J., Levo Y., et al.: Mixed cryoglobulinemia: Clinical aspects and long-term follow-up of 40 patients. *Am. J. Med.* 69:287, 1980.
146. Tarantino A., De Vecchi A., Montagnino G., et al.: Renal disease in essential mixed cryoglobulinemia. *Q. J. Med.* 50:1, 1981.
147. Meadow S.R., Glasgow E.F., White R.H.R.: Schonlein-Henoch nephritis. *Q. J. Med.* 41:241, 1972.
148. Travers R.L., Allison D.J., Brattle R.P., et al.: Polyarteritis nodosa: a clinical and angiographic analysis of 17 cases. *Semin. Arthritis Rheum.* 8:184, 1979.
149. Felts J.H.: Hereditary nephritis with the nephrotic syndrome. *Arch. Intern. Med.* 125:459, 1970.
150. Chazan J.A., Zacks J., Cohen J.J., et al.: Hereditary nephritis: clinical spectrum and mode of inheritance in five new kindreds. *Am. J. Med.* 50:764, 1971.
151. Cheigh J.S., Mouradian J., Scisin M., et al.: Kidney transplant nephrotic syndrome: Relationship between allograft histopathology and natural course. *Kidney Int.* 18:358, 1980.
152. Torres V.E., Velosa J.A., Holley K.E., et al.: The progression of vesicoureteral reflux nephropathy. *Ann. Intern. Med.* 92:776, 1980.
153. Cotran R.S.: Glomerulosclerosis in reflux nephropathy. *Kidney Int.* 21:528, 1982.
154. Kumar A., Shapiro A.P.: Proteinuria and nephrotic syndrome induced by renin in patients with renal artery stenosis. *Arch. Intern. Med.* 140:1631, 1980.

5 Idiopathic Nephrotic Syndrome

HEAVY PROTEINURIA in the absence of systemic illness or obvious etiologic associations is designated as the idiopathic nephrotic syndrome (INS). Virtually all primary glomerular diseases can be accompanied by heavy proteinuria, but only four glomerulopathies comprise 90% of all cases of INS (Table 5–1). In many instances, clinical characteristics including age at onset and the presence or absence of hypertension, hematuria, or renal insufficiency will suggest the correct etiologic diagnosis. However, precise diagnosis and formulation of a rational therapeutic approach often require histologic examination of renal tissue. In this chapter we focus on the salient pathologic and clinical features of membranous glomerulopathy, minimal change disease, focal glomerular sclerosis, and membranoproliferative glomerulonephritis.

MEMBRANOUS GLOMERULOPATHY

Epidemiology

Membranous glomerulopathy (MGN) accounts for approximately 40% of adult cases of INS but less than 10% of pediatric cases.[1-3] Age at the time of clinical onset ranges from 2 to 75 years with an average age of 40. The relatively frequent association of MGN with neoplasia in adults is not found in pediatric series.[4] For unknown reasons, males outnumber females by a ratio of approximately 2:1.

Pathology

Characteristic light microscopic changes in idiopathic MGN include diffuse uniform thickening of the glomerular basement membrane

TABLE 5–1.—CLINICAL FEATURES OF ADULT IDIOPATHIC NEPHROTIC SYNDROME

HISTOLOGY	% OF ADULT INS	AVERAGE AGE AT ONSET	CLINICAL FINDINGS AT DIAGNOSIS*			
			Nephrotic Syndrome	Hypertension	Hematuria	Decreased GFR
Membranous glomerulopathy	40	40–50	75	25	60	25
Minimal change disease	20	30–40	100	5	20	5–10
Focal glomerular sclerosis	20	35–45	45	40	70	25
Membranoproliferative glomerulonephritis	10	25–35	50	40	90	60
Other†	10	—	—	—	—	—

*Values are given as percentages derived from a review of the literature.
†Includes unclassified proliferative lesions.

(GBM), mild expansion of the mesangial matrix, and little or no increase in mesangial cellularity. Depending on the stage of the disease, however, a spectrum of histologic findings ranging from essentially normal-appearing glomeruli on light microscopy to marked thickening of the GBM and early glomerular sclerosis may be seen (Fig 5–1). Special silver impregnation techniques reveal characteristic subepithelial "spikes" consisting of basement membrane projections between adjacent subepithelial immune-deposits (Fig 5–2).[3, 5] Significant mesangial hypercellularity is unusual and, when observed, should raise suspicion of membranous nephropathy of SLE. Tubulointerstitial changes are not prominent early in the course of idiopathic MGN, but interstitial edema, interstitial fibrosis, and tubular atrophy may develop as the disease progresses.

Immunofluorescence microscopy demonstrates a characteristic granular subepithelial staining for IgG in all cases of idiopathic MGN; C3 is found in a similar distribution in approximately 75% of cases and IgA and IgM in less than one third.[3, 6] Prominent staining for IgA and IgM suggests lupus nephritis, especially when associated with mesangial immune-deposits. Although light and immunofluorescence microscopic findings are often sufficiently characteristic to suggest the diagnosis of MGN, electron microscopic examination is the most accurate method of identifying MGN, particularly when light microscopic findings are equivocal (Fig 5–3). Ultrastructural examination of renal tissue usually reveals electron-dense deposits in the subepithelial portion of the GBM. Typically, mesangial deposits are not found. In histologically advanced cases, the initially discrete sub-

Idiopathic Nephrotic Syndrome

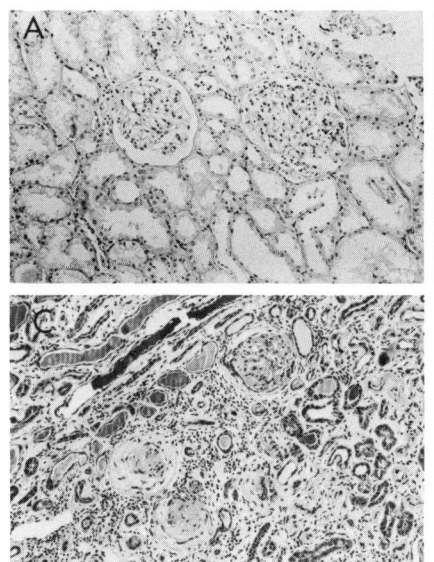

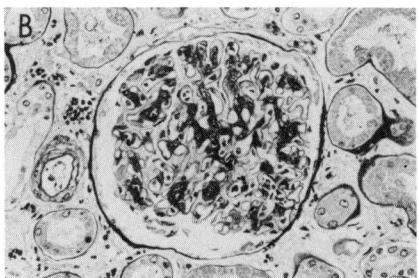

Fig 5–1.—The histologic spectrum of isiopathic membranous glomerulopathy. **A,** hematoxylin and eosin-stained section with essentially normal glomerular architecture. Electron microscopy, however, revealed characteristic subepithelial electron dense deposits. **B,** periodic acid-Schiff-stained biopsy specimen demonstrating moderate mesangial expansion and thickened capillary loops. **C,** hematoxylin and eosin stain of a renal biopsy with advanced membranous nephropathy. The GBM is markedly widened and two glomeruli demonstrate early sclerosis.

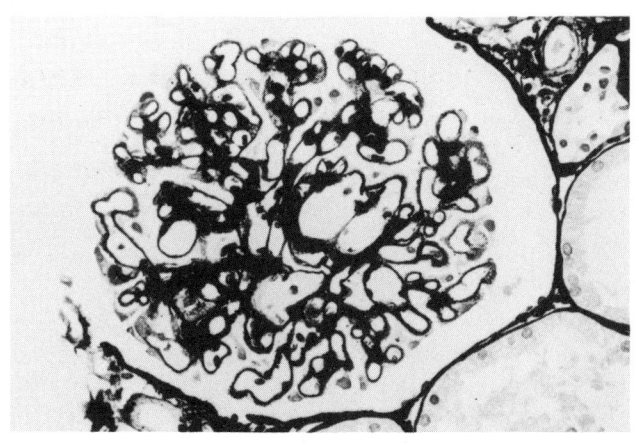

Fig 5–2.—Silver stain of a glomerulus with membranous glomerulopathy. Capillary loops sectioned at right angles show the characteristic subepithelial spikes whereas those cut tangentially demonstrate a "moth-eaten" appearance.

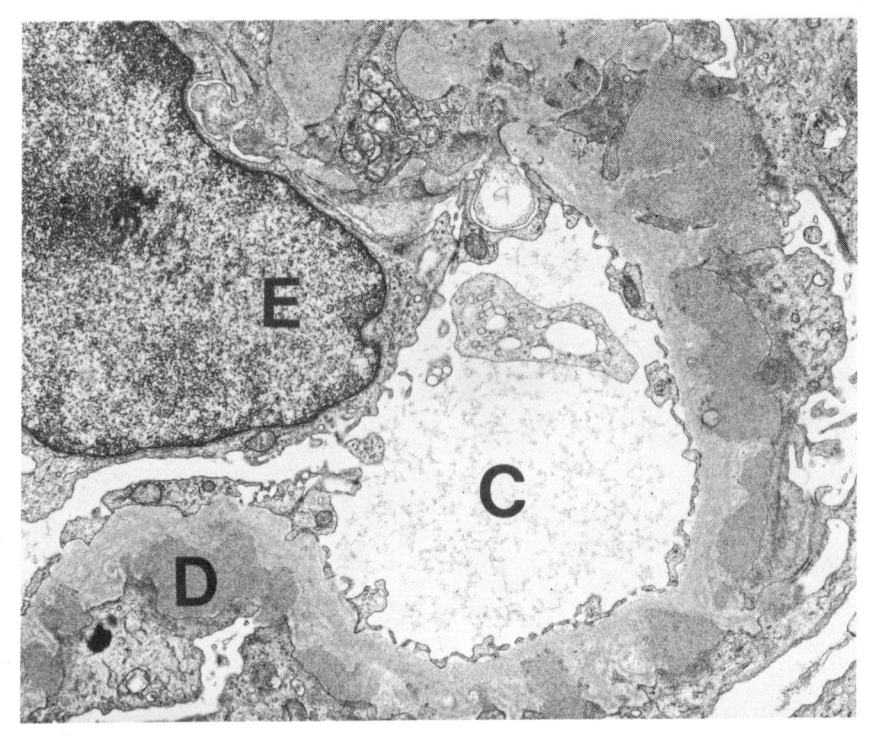

Fig 5–3.—Electron micrograph of a capillary loop from a biopsy specimen with idiopathic membranous glomerulopathy. There are multiple discreet subepithelial electron dense deposits *(D)* characteristic of membranous nephropathy. Capillary lumen *(C)*; endothelial cell *(E)*.

epithelial deposits may evolve to large, electron-dense intramembranous deposits and finally to electron-lucent intramembranous deposits.[5,7] Histologic staging based on such ultrastructural alterations does not correspond precisely to the clinical stage of MGN; renal function is more closely correlated with the accompanying tubulointerstitial disease.

Pathogenesis

During the past two decades, extensive investigations of the pathogenesis of both experimental and human MGN have focused on the immunologic abnormalities fundamental to this disorder and on the mechanisms by which immune-complexes are deposited in the glomerulus. An exhaustive review of these investigations is beyond the scope of this chapter (see Chapter 2); however, a limited discussion of the major hypotheses regarding the pathogenesis of MGN is relevant. Although antigen-antibody systems accounting for immune-complex deposition have been identified in many secondary forms of MGN (see Chapter 4 and Table 6–2), the responsible antigenic stimulus in idiopathic MGN is unknown.[6, 8] The histologic similarity between Heymann nephritis in the rat and human idiopathic MGN led to initial speculation that an abnormal antibody response to renal tubular epithelial antigen (RTE) might be responsible for immune-complex deposition in MGN. Occasional reports suggest that the RTE-anti-RTE system might play a role in isolated cases; however, there is little evidence for its participation in the majority of patients with idiopathic MGN.[8–10] Zager and co-workers were unable to document the presence of circulating anti-RTE antibody in any of 29 patients with idiopathic MGN.[8] Other work has suggested that immune-complex glomerulonephritis in general, and MGN in particular, might be the result of an immunologic deficiency rather than enhanced antibody synthesis.[11, 12] For example, Ooi et al. have shown that monocytes from patients with idiopathic MGN inhibit IgG and IgM synthesis by both autologous and heterologous lymphocytes. These workers theorized that reduced antibody synthesis impairs antigenic clearance, and accounts for immune-complex formation either through deposition of circulating complexes or through in situ complex formation.[12]

Many former concepts regarding the pathogenesis of human MGN were drawn by analogy from experimental models of chronic serum sickness which suggested that localization of immune-deposits was chiefly dependent on the size and avidity of circulating complexes (Chapter 2). In serum sickness models, small immune-complexes formed in zones of antigen excess or with low-avidity antibody readily penetrate the GBM and deposit in the subepithelial space.[3, 6, 13] By analogy, human MGN was believed to result from the subepithelial deposition of *circulating* immune-complexes. However, the failure to detect circulating complexes in the majority of patients with MGN[6, 8] prompted experimental studies that have revised this concept. Recent work provides strong support for the theory that MGN results from the interaction of circulating antibody with local GBM antigens or circulating antigens that have become fixed in the GBM.[3, 13] The anionic composition of the GBM is an important determinant in this localization process. Cationic antigens or positively charged complexes tend to localize in the negatively charged subepithelial space and elicit a subsequent antibody response.[13–15] The binding of free antibody to these planted antigens results in in situ immune-complex formation. While the exact antigenic stimulus in idiopathic MGN remains undefined, it is likely that impaired clearance of cationic antigens or possibly small molecular weight complexes results in subepithelial immune-deposits. These deposits then induce the release of secondary reactants that alter both the size and charge-selectivity of the GBM, leading to heavy nonselective proteinuria.

Clinical Features

The clinical features of MGN have been well documented in several large series (Table 5–1).[1, 2, 7, 16] In adults, the average age of clinical onset is between 40 and 50 years. Heavy proteinuria is present at the time of diagnosis in approximately 70% of cases and the frank nephrotic syndrome ultimately develops in 80%.[1–3, 16] One quarter of patients with histologically proved MGN, however, have only mild to moderate proteinuria. Microscopic hematuria occurs in over 50% but gross hematuria is rare. Hypertension and renal insufficiency (serum creatinine >1.5 mg/dl) are present in 25% of cases at the time of diagnosis. Circulating immune-complexes are detectable in less than one third of cases and complement levels are normal in virtually all.[1, 3, 8]

There are two noteworthy associations among patients with MGN: neoplasia and renal vein thrombosis. Solid neoplasms occur in approximately 10% of adults with MGN but are rare in children (Chapter 4).[1, 4] In the adult population, carcinoma of the lung, colon, and breast are the most common solid tumors linked to MGN. The development of apparently idiopathic MGN in adults, especially after the age of 60, should thus alert the physician to the possibility of an underlying neoplasm. Although hypercoagulability is a nonspecific consequence of heavy proteinuria (Chapter 3), MGN appears to be overrepresented among patients with the nephrotic syndrome and renal vein thrombosis. Some studies suggest that as many as 30% to 50% of patients with MGN and the nephrotic syndrome have renal vein thrombosis,[16–18] but the diagnostic and therapeutic implications of these findings are not well defined. Because renal venography and long-term anticoagulation therapy are not without hazard, our policy has been to limit diagnostic and therapeutic maneuvers to patients with symptomatic thromboembolism.

The clinical course of MGN has been carefully documented in a number of long-term studies.[1, 2, 7, 16] Some of these reports include patients treated with corticosteroids, but the doses employed were relatively modest and no appreciable effect of steroid therapy was noted.[1, 2, 7] If these studies are combined with the results of a recent investigation of over 100 untreated patients,[16] a well-defined picture of the natural history of MGN emerges. Within five years from the time of diagnosis, 25% of patients progress to end-stage renal disease (ESRD), 50% demonstrate persistent nephrotic syndrome or moderate proteinuria, and 25% undergo a spontaneous complete remission. During the ensuing years an increasing proportion of patients progress to ESRD; by 15 years approximately 40% have developed terminal renal failure (Fig 5–4). Most investigators agree that renal failure occurs with substantially greater frequency in patients with the nephrotic syndrome compared to those with lesser amounts of proteinuria, and that spontaneous remissions are more common in subjects with well-preserved GFR at the time of diagnosis.[1, 2, 19]

Therapy

Most, but not all, uncontrolled studies of MGN have shown little benefit of corticosteroid or cytotoxic drug therapy.[1–3, 5] In addition, several controlled studies utilizing low-dose steroid (30 mg of predni-

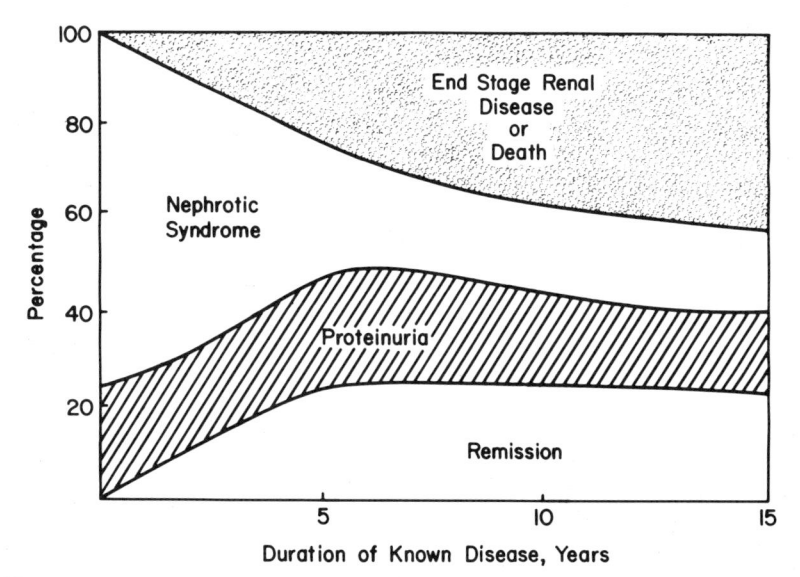

Fig 5–4.—Estimated long-term course of adults with MGN. Within five years of diagnosis, approximately equal percentages of patients undergo spontaneous complete remission, exhibit moderate proteinuria, persist with the nephrotic syndrome, or progress to ESRD. After 15 years, 40% have developed terminal renal failure. (Modified with permission from Cameron J.S.: *Kidney Int.* 15:88, 1979.)

sone daily or less) or cytotoxic drug regimens have not demonstrated a beneficial effect in the treated groups.[20-22] However, two recently conducted, controlled studies suggest substantial benefit from corticosteroid or immunosuppressive therapy or both. Coggins and co-workers randomly assigned adult patients with well-preserved renal function and the nephrotic syndrome due to idiopathic MGN to receive either high-dose, alternate day prednisone (average 125 mg q.o.d.) or placebo.[23] After an average follow-up period of two years, they noted a significant increase in the rate of complete or partial remissions in the treated group. More importantly, the group receiving prednisone exhibited significantly better preservation of renal function; GFR declined by an average of 10% per year in the placebo group but only by 2% per year in the treated patients. Over the period of observation, 11 of 38 patients in the control group sustained a twofold or greater increase in serum creatinine compared to only 2 of 34 in the treated group. These authors and others have suggested that short-term, alternate day prednisone treatment exerts a beneficial effect on the ultimate course of MGN.[23, 24] In a more recent randomized study, Ponticelli and colleagues demonstrated that methylprednisolone and chlorambucil, administered for six months, resulted in significantly more remissions and better preservation of GFR compared to placebo treatment.[25]

Taken together, the available data support the use of short-term corticosteroid or cytotoxic therapy in patients with idiopathic MGN and the nephrotic syndrome. It has been our practice to treat patients with biopsy-proven MGN with high-dose, alternate day prednisone (125 mg q.o.d.) for two months, followed by gradual tapering and discontinuation of steroids over an additional two-month period. This regimen is associated with few adverse reactions and is as effective as combined regimens that include cytotoxic agents with potentially hazardous long-term consequences. In patients who respond with a complete remission,* repeated courses of steroids are given only for relapses of symptomatic nephrotic syndrome. Patients with a sustained partial remission have an excellent long-term prognosis and require no further steroid therapy.

Patients who develop chronic renal failure due to MGN are candidates for dialysis and transplantation according to the same criteria applicable to the general population with ESRD. Unlike some other glomerulopathies associated with idiopathic nephrotic syndrome, MGN rarely recurs in renal allografts.

---

*Complete remission is defined as the excretion of less than 150 mg of protein per day. Partial remission is the excretion of 150 mg to 2,000 mg of protein daily.

MINIMAL CHANGE DISEASE

Epidemiology

Minimal change disease (MCD) accounts for approximately 20% of all cases of adult INS (Table 5–1).[26, 27] This disorder, also known as *lipoid nephrosis* or *nil disease,* is the most common cause of INS in childhood but decreases in prevalence with increasing age. In most series, males outnumber females by a ratio of 2:1.[26, 28–36]

Pathology

The glomeruli appear normal by light microscopy in MCD. Interstitial edema, consequent to hypoalbuminemia, and vacuolization of proximal tubular cells, due to reabsorption of filtered lipoproteins, are frequent but nonspecific findings. The only characteristic histologic change is found on ultrastructural examination; apparent "fusion" or effacement of the epithelial foot processes is a constant feature on electron microscopy (Fig 5–5). This finding, related to loss of electrostatic charge, is observed in virtually all glomerular diseases accompanied by heavy proteinuria and is not pathognomonic of MCD. Electron-dense deposits are conspicuously absent. Immunofluorescent staining is negative for immunoglobulins and complement.

Many investigators have described patients who are clinically indistinguishable from subjects with classical MCD but exhibit mild degrees of mesangial cell proliferation or positive mesangial immunofluorescence staining for IgM.[27, 37–39] Whether these patients represent a distinct entity or part of a spectrum that includes MCD requires further investigation. Further broadening of histologic criteria to include more severe degrees of mesangial proliferation or areas of segmental glomerular sclerosis alters clinicopathologic correlations, resulting in increased incidence of steroid resistance and progression to renal failure.[27–28] Because the relationships between MCD, mesangioproliferative glomerulonephritis, and focal glomerular sclerosis are not firmly established, we prefer a more restricted histologic definition.

Pathogenesis

The exact pathogenesis of MCD is unknown. Although histologic changes clearly indicate that the disorder is not an immune-complex

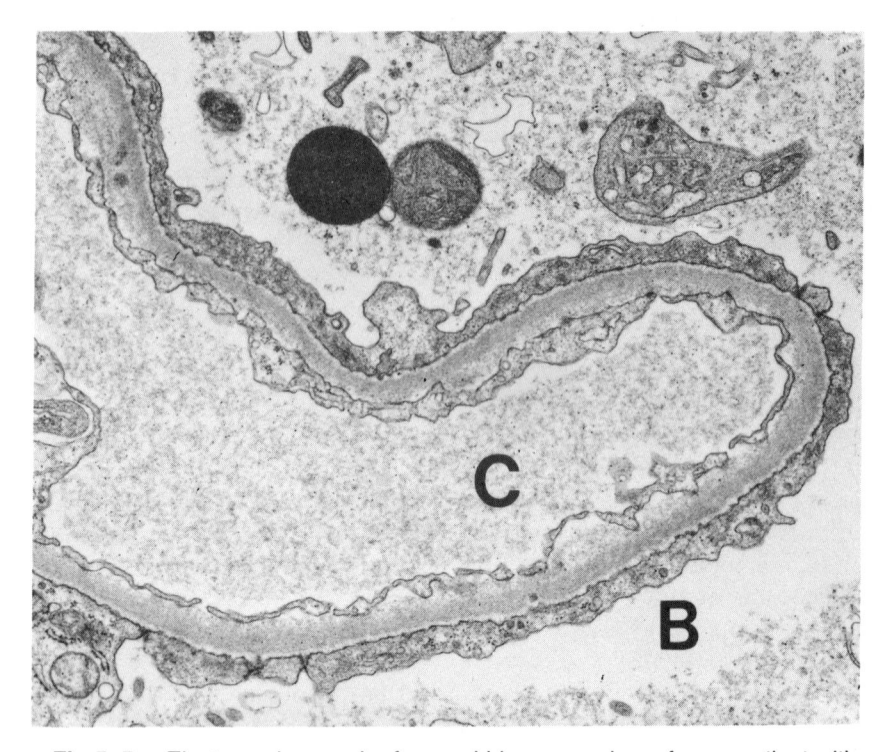

Fig 5–5.—Electron micrograph of a renal biopsy specimen from a patient with minimal change disease. The only abnormality is a diffuse spreading or "fusion" of the epithelial foot processes over the GBM. Capillary lumen *(C);* Bowman's space *(B)*.

glomerulopathy in the strict sense, several indirect lines of evidence support the concept that MCD is immunologically mediated. First, the association of Hodgkin's disease with some cases of MCD implies an etiologic relation (see Chapter 4). Because Hodgkin's disease is a disorder of T lymphocytes, some workers have speculated that a lymphokine produced by normal T-cells might alter glomerular permselectivity, but direct proof is lacking.[40, 41] Reduced levels of IgG and IgA and increased concentrations of IgM in the sera of patients with MCD may also reflect T-cell dysfunctions.[42] Moreover, Nagata and coworkers have recently demonstrated an increased number of infiltrating T-cells in the glomeruli of subjects with MCD.[43] Finally, measles infection, known to suppress T-cell function, has been linked to remissions of the nephrotic syndrome in MCD.[27] Another line of evidence derives from the clear-cut, but poorly understood relation between atopy and MCD. The incidence of atopic disease appears to be increased in children with MCD and the disorder has been precipitated occasionally by hypersensitivity reactions, suggesting an allergic basis in some cases.[27, 44] The most persuasive evidence regarding an immunologic basis for MCD stems from its rapid response to immunosuppressive therapy with corticosteroids and/or cytotoxic drugs.

While the proximate cause of MCD remains obscure, recent work by Myers and associates has characterized the defect in glomerular permselectivity. Utilizing both a mathematical model and clinical studies which examined the filtration of neutral dextrans, these investigators have concluded that proteinuria in MCD results from a defect in the electrostatic barrier function of the GBM.[45, 46] The bulk of evidence thus suggests that, in MCD, a poorly characterized immunologic abnormality, possibly related to T-cell dysfunction, directly alters glomerular permselectivity. Heavy proteinuria results from a loss of the normal anionic charge of the GBM and not from a size-selective defect in the glomerular filtration barrier.

Clinical Features

The clinical manifestations of MCD are those of the prototypical nephrotic syndrome. Peak onset in adults is between the ages of 30 and 40 and heavy proteinuria is present in all patients at the time of diagnosis (Table 5–1). Urinary protein excretion ranges from 3.5 to more than 20 gm per day and is often greater than 10 gm.[26, 27, 30, 47] Hypoalbuminemia and its consequences including dependent edema, anasarca, and hypercholesterolemia are present in most subjects. When serum albumin concentrations are reduced below 2.0 gm/dl, spontaneous pleural effusions, pulmonary edema, and ascites can occur. Total hemolytic complement and C3 and C4 levels are normal in virtually all patients with MCD.[27]

In contrast to other causes of INS, hypertension, hematuria, and renal insufficiency are rare. Microscopic hematuria is present in less than 20% of cases, while hypertension and azotemia occur in less than 5% and 10%, respectively. When renal insufficiency occurs, it is generally mild and readily reversible with remission of the nephrotic syndrome. However, several recent reports have documented the occurrence of acute renal failure in adults with MCD.[32, 33, 48] In some of these cases the renal insufficiency has been irreversible, but in the majority renal function normalized with the natriuresis induced by the administration of diuretics or steroid therapy (Fig 5–6). These

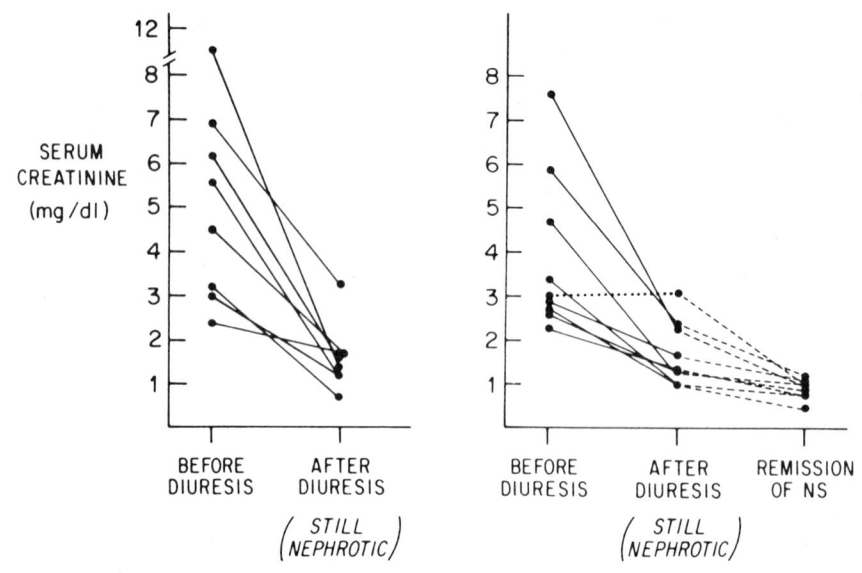

Fig 5–6.—Reversal of renal insufficiency in response to diuresis in patients with steroid-resistant *(left panel)* and steroid-responsive *(right panel)* MCD. (Courtesy of Lowenstein J., et al.: *Am. J. Med.* 70:227, 1981.)

observations, along with the finding of a disproportionate reduction in GFR compared to renal blood flow, have suggested that acute renal failure may result from increased intratubular pressure consequent to interstitial edema.[33] Whatever the exact mechanism, the phenomenon of reversible renal failure in a subset of patients with MCD is noteworthy and underscores the fact that the mere presence of azotemia in adults with INS does not preclude an excellent outcome. The proclivity of patients with INS, especially MCD, to develop serious infections was fully discussed in Chapter 3. Since the advent of antimicrobial and steroid therapy in the early 1950s, the incidence of life-threatening infections has declined markedly. Nevertheless, in untreated patients, the decreased serum levels of IgG and Factor B greatly increase the risk of infection with encapsulated bacteria.[27] With steroid-induced or spontaneous remissions, Factor B levels normalize whereas IgG concentrations increase toward, but not entirely to, normal.[42]

Therapy

Since MCD is more prevalent in children than adults, most of our knowledge concerning the natural history, response to therapy, and long-term outcome of this disorder is derived from the pediatric literature [26-28, 34-36, 49, 50]; however, observations in children are generally applicable to adults. Although a controlled clinical trial examining the benefits of steroid therapy in MCD has never been conducted, the therapeutic efficacy of corticosteroids is widely acknowledged. Most investigators agree that short-term treatment with prednisone (1 mg/kg/day or 2 mg/kg q.o.d.) reduces morbidity and mortality and increases the rate of remission. With this regimen, 90% of children and approximately 50% of adults achieve a complete remission within four weeks. After eight weeks of therapy, 90% of adults with biopsy-proven MCD no longer exhibit proteinuria.[49] Whether the more rapid response in children is due to the relatively higher doses of steroids employed in pediatric series (60 mg/M^2/day) or other identified factors is unclear.

Approximately one quarter of all patients with MCD achieve a lasting remission after an initial course of steroids (Figure 5–7).[26, 27, 50, 51] Twenty percent develop infrequent relapses of the nephrotic syndrome that respond promptly to repeat corticosteroid therapy. An additional 20% exhibit multiple relapses with nephrotic range proteinuria returning shortly after steroids are discontinued. Twenty-five percent of subjects with MCD exhibit steroid dependency, i.e., recurrence of proteinuria whenever the steroid regimen is tapered. Ten percent or less have continued nephrotic range proteinuria despite steroid therapy. Moreover, renal biopsies of patients with steroid resistance often reveal evidence of focal glomerular sclerosis, even when earlier biopsies have suggested MCD. The long-term prognosis in this steroid-resistant group of patients is poorer than in steroid-responsive subjects and includes a relatively high rate of progression

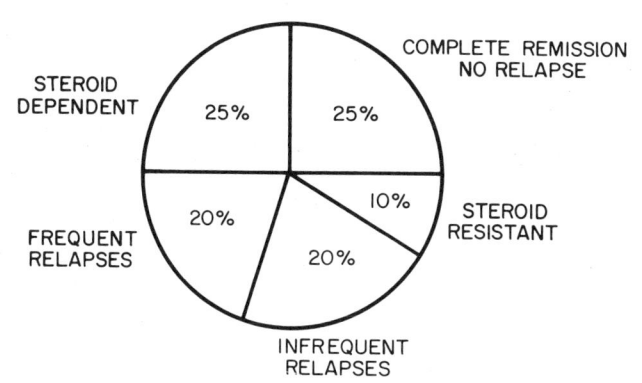

Fig 5–7.—Approximate response to corticosteroid therapy in MCD.[26, 27, 50, 51]

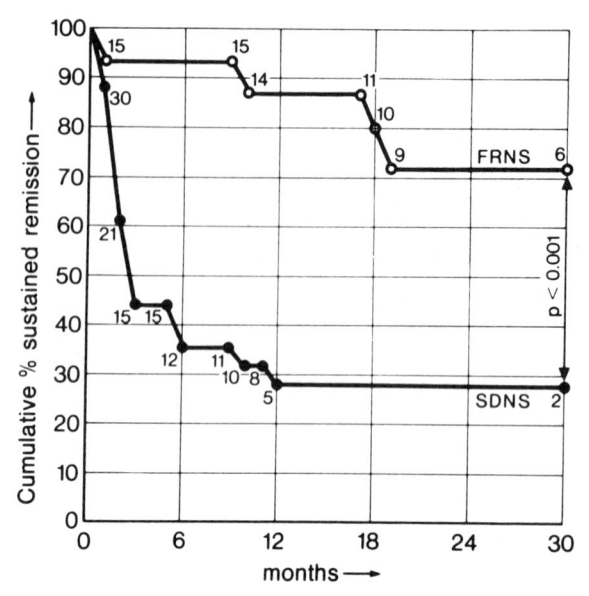

Fig 5–8.—Cumulative percentage of sustained remissions in response to cytotoxic drug therapy in children with frequently relapsing nephrotic syndrome *(FRNS)* and those with steroid-dependent nephrotic syndrome *(SDNS)*. (Courtesy of *N. Engl. J. Med.* 306:451, 1982.)

to renal insufficiency. Because focal sclerosis frequently begins in the corticomedullary region (see below), sampling error may account for the failure to detect glomerular sclerosis early in the course of the disease.[26, 27]

The beneficial effect of cytotoxic drug therapy in patients with frequently relapsing or steroid-dependent MCD has been documented in several studies.[28, 34–36, 51, 52] Both cyclophosphamide (2 mg/kg/day) and chlorambucil (0.15 to 0.20 mg/kg/day), given in combination with prednisone over an eight-week course, result in an increased rate of sustained remissions in both groups.[28, 34–36] Most workers agree that the overall response to cytotoxic drug therapy is better in patients with frequently relapsing MCD than in those with the steroid-dependent variety (Fig 5–8).[27, 34] Despite recent work suggesting that short-term, low-dose cyclophosphamide therapy is devoid of lasting effects on immune function, cytotoxic drugs should be used with caution.[36, 51, 52] We reserve cytotoxic therapy for patients who develop intolerable side effects from corticosteroid treatment such as severe hypertension, diabetes, or psychiatric dysfunction.

As we have already indicated, a small percentage of patients with

MCD (less than 2% to 3%) ultimately progress to renal insufficiency. These subjects are atypical, however, since the prognosis is excellent in the vast majority. In general, the natural tendency of MCD is for an increasing percentage of patients to undergo remission with time. After a disease-free interval of three or more years, recurrence of MCD is distinctly unusual.[53] Pru and co-workers, however, recently reported a late recurrence rate of 4% in a series of 400 patients with MCD.[31] In most, repeat biopsy revealed MCD and the clinical course and response to therapy were similar to the initial episodes of disease.

FOCAL GLOMERULAR SCLEROSIS

Epidemiology

Focal glomerular sclerosis (FGS) or focal segmental glomerulosclerosis refers to a histologic pattern of renal injury that can result from a primary disorder or consequent to a variety of glomerular, tubulointerstitial, or vascular diseases. Secondary forms of FGS are uncommon causes of the nephrotic syndrome, but primary FGS accounts for approximately 10% of pediatric cases and 20% of adult cases of INS.[54, 55] In adults, the clinical onset of idiopathic FGS occurs between the ages of 20 to 70 years with a median age of 35 (Table 5–1). In contrast to membranous glomerulopathy and minimal change disease (MCD) in which males predominate, in FGS males and females are affected equally.[54–57]

Pathology

Idiopathic FGS is characterized by a spectrum of histologic changes. Typically, light microscopy reveals focal (some but not all glomeruli) and segmental (only a portion of the glomerulus) glomerular sclerosis (Fig 5–9). Involved glomeruli often demonstrate an increase in mesangial matrix that is most prominent at the vascular pole.[55, 58] Wrinkling of the GBM and collapse of capillary loops are frequent and are best demonstrated by periodic acid-Schiff (PAS) or silver stains. Mesangial cellularity is generally normal but in some cases may be mildly increased. Focal areas of tubular atrophy and interstitial fibrosis are characteristic and at times may seem out of proportion to glomerular disease.[54, 55, 58] Early studies of FGS emphasized the fact that juxtamedullary glomeruli are primarily involved with relative sparing outer cortical glomeruli in early stages of the disease. Most, but not all, subsequent reports have confirmed this predilection for initial juxtamedullary involvement.[54, 57] Consequently, when a limited sample of superficial renal cortex is obtained by percutaneous renal biopsy in a patient with heavy proteinuria, the presence of significant tubulointerstitial disease with minimal glomerular abnormalities should suggest FGS.

Approximately 80% of cases of FGS demonstrate the characteristic focal, segmental histologic pattern. A minority, however, reveal a peculiar form of global glomerular sclerosis.[55, 58, 59] Light microscopy shows focal areas of interstitial fibrosis and totally sclerotic glomeruli interspersed among apparently normal glomeruli (Fig 5–9). In this variety of FGS, intermediate histologic stages between globally sclerotic and normal glomeruli are not seen.

Several patterns of immunofluoresence have been described in FGS.[54–58] The most common occurs in two thirds of patients and is characterized by a coarse granular staining for IgM and C3 in the sclerotic tufts; occasionally, IgG or IgA are found in a similar distribution. Nonsclerotic glomeruli usually do not exhibit deposition of immunoglobulins or complement. In some cases, a weak linear staining for IgM and C3 is demonstrated along the GBM. One group of investigators has described a linear deposition of IgG in glomerular capillary loops in adults with FGS and nephrotic syndrome.[60] This latter pattern is distinctly unusual, however, and may represent a form of heroin-associated nephropathy (see Chapter 4).

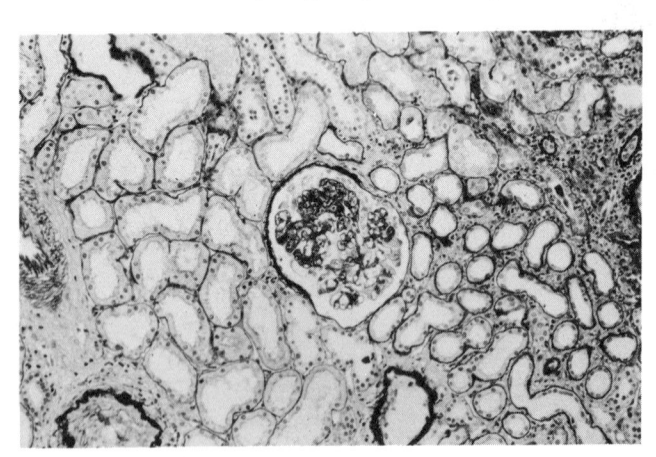

Fig 5–9.—Periodic acid-Schiff stain of a renal biopsy with focal segmental glomerulosclerosis. The glomerulus shows an area of segmental sclerosis with an increase in mesangial matrix and collapse of capillary loops.

Electron microscopy in FGS confirms the light microscopic findings. Except for occasional paramesangial or subendothelial electron-dense deposits, ultrastructural evidence of an immune-complex nephropathy is notably lacking.[54, 55, 57, 58] In patients with nephrotic range proteinuria, effacement of epithelial foot processes is characteristic and is found even in nonsclerotic glomeruli.

Pathogenesis

During the past decade, there has been intense investigation and considerable speculation regarding the pathogenesis of FGS. Controversies concerning the pathogenesis of FGS revolve around two key issues: 1) the relationship of FGS to both MCD and mesangioproliferative glomerulonephritis, and 2) the role of hemodynamic factors in the development of the glomerular sclerosis and consequent proteinuria.

Debate regarding the relation of FGS to MCD has continued since Rich's original description of FGS in 1957.[61] One school of thought considers FGS, MCD, and mesangioproliferative glomerulonephritis as interrelated diseases along a histologic continuum. There are several arguments which support this hypothesis.[54–56] Some patients with histologically documented MCD have demonstrated clear-cut FGS on subsequent renal biopsy. In addition, the clinical features and the initial response to immunosuppressive therapy in the three disorders are frequently indistinguishable. Finally, there are often similar immunofluorescence and electron microscopic findings in MCD, mesangioproliferative glomerulonephritis, and the nonsclerotic glomeruli of FGS. These lines of evidence are suggestive, but they do not prove that the three diseases are related. By contrast, the observation of sclerotic glomeruli early in the course of the INS, the nonselective pattern of urinary protein excretion in FGS, and its poorer response to cytotoxic drugs have led some investigators to conclude that FGS and MCD, at least, are distinct entities.

The recent interest in nonimmunologically mediated mechanisms of proteinuria, particularly the effects of glomerular hyperperfusion on renal histology and protein excretion, has suggested to some that FGS may be hemodynamically mediated. A large body of experimental and clinical evidence (see Chapter 2) exists to support the concept that, in both animals and man, progressive ablation of renal tissue results in an increased GFR in remnant nephrons. Glomerular hyperfiltration increases proteinuria and leads to eventual sclerosis of residual glomeruli. This mechanism has been postulated to account for secondary FGS in some cases of poststreptococcal glomerulonephritis, chronic allograft rejection, reflux nephropathy, and analgesic abuse nephropathy.[54,55] In addition, the observation that juxtamedullary nephrons have an increased GFR compared to cortical nephrons, lends credence to the role of hemodynamic factors in the pathogenesis of idiopathic FGS.[56] But pathogenetic mechanisms involved in secondary FGS should be applied cautiously, if at all, to primary FGS. Most patients with histologically documented FGS have normal or nearly normal GFRs at the time of diagnosis, making it unlikely that a reduction in renal mass has caused the glomerular sclerosis. Further, even nonsclerotic glomeruli demonstrate histologic evidence of heavy proteinuria (effacement of epithelial foot processes), implying a more subtle biochemical abnormality. Finally, the rapid recurrence of heavy proteinuria and glomerular sclerosis in some patients within days of renal transplantation suggests a humoral mechanism. Thus, although hemodynamic alterations are likely to be pathogenetically involved in secondary FGS, there is little firm evidence that they play a role in primary FGS.

Clinical Features

Some of the relevant clinical manifestations of FGS are shown in Table 5-1. The nephrotic syndrome is a cardinal feature of FGS and is present in an average of 45% of patients at the outset of the disease and in as many as 60% at some time during their course.[54-57] However, studies which have not restricted renal biopsy to patients with heavy proteinuria, suggest that as few as one third of subjects with histologically diagnosed FGS develop the nephrotic syndrome.[59] Hypertension is present in 40% when FGS is first diagnosed, and microscopic hematuria is found in 70% of cases. Reduced renal function is present in one quarter of patients at the outset. There are no consistent serologic abnormalities in FGS; complement levels are normal and circulating immune-complexes are absent. Although most studies suggest that pregnancy does not exert an especially deleterious effect on any single histologic type of renal disease, one recent report noted a particularly adverse effect of pregnancy on the course of FGS.[61]

The long-term course of FGS has been well documented in both the pediatric and adult literature.[54-59,63] Most investigators agree that the nephrotic syndrome develops in all children with FGS at some time during the course of the disease.[57,63] In contrast, heavy proteinuria is not invariable in the adult population with FGS. Moreover, in adults, but not in children, the nephrotic syndrome predicts a high rate of progression to ESRD.[54, 55, 59, 63]

The exact incidence of spontaneous remission in FGS is difficult to estimate but approximates 10%. Another 10% of patients experience a rapid progression to ESRD within one to three years of diagnosis. Ten years after the onset, one half of adult patients develop ESRD; renal failure occurs in 50% of children after 15 years.[54, 55, 58, 63] The remainder of subjects with FGS exhibit persistent proteinuria, hypertension, and variable degrees of renal insufficiency.

Therapy

Prospective controlled trials investigating the efficacy of corticosteroid or cytotoxic drug therapy in FGS have not been published. Multiple uncontrolled studies have reported a 10% to 20% rate of complete remission and a 40% to 50% incidence of partial remission in response to steroid therapy.[26, 54–58, 63] In addition, there is general agreement that the long-term course of the disease is unaltered even if urinary protein excretion is reduced by corticosteroids. We do not uniformly advocate steroid therapy in biopsy-proven FGS.

The influence of cytotoxic drugs on the course of histologically documented FGS is equally unsettled. A recent retrospective study suggested that a partial response to cyclophosphamide predicted a reduced rate of progression to ESRD in children with steroid-resistant FGS.[64] However, further investigation, especially in adults, is required before the role of cytotoxic therapy in FGS is firmly established.

Based on these limited data, it is difficult to formulate a rational therapeutic approach to FGS. We prefer to individualize steroid therapy in each case depending on the duration of disease, age, and the presence or absence of nephrotic range proteinuria. We do not employ cytotoxic drugs in adults with steroid-resistant FGS; however, pediatric patients should be considered candidates for cytotoxic drug therapy.

Since a large percentage of patients with FGS eventually develop ESRD, the treatment of this segment of the population with chronic renal insufficiency has been carefully studied. Although long-term survival is not different in patients with FGS compared to the general population with ESRD, the documented rate of recurrence in renal allografts is the highest of any primary glomerulopathy. Overall, FGS recurs in approximately one third of all renal transplants.[54, 55, 58, 65–67] Several studies suggest that, in the rapidly progressive form of the disease, this incidence approaches 50%.[54, 66, 67] It would seem prudent to restrict live, related donor allografts to patients with the more indolent form of FGS.

MEMBRANOPROLIFERATIVE GLOMERULONEPHRITIS

Epidemiology

Membranoproliferative glomerulonephritis (MPGN) accounts for approximately 10% of both pediatric and adult cases of INS. The disease has been classified into Type I and Type II varieties on the basis of renal histology. The more prevalent Type I MPGN occurs at a mean age of 30, whereas Type II MPGN is more frequent in the pediatric population, with a mean age of onset of approximately 20 years.[68, 69] Males and females are equally affected.

Pathology

Although there are a few clinical differences between the two types of MPGN, the only clear distinction is derived from histologic examination of renal tissue. Type I disease accounts for approximately 70% of all cases of MPGN.[68–72] The histologic pattern in idiopathic Type I MPGN is not pathognomonic and can be found in association with other disorders such as hepatitis B, SLE, and sickle cell disease (Chapter 4 and Table 6–2).[72, 73] The histologic findings in Type II MPGN are unique and, with the exception of lipodystrophy, have not been described in association with systemic disease. Secondary forms of MPGN must be excluded on clinical grounds and by appropriate laboratory studies before a diagnosis of idiopathic MPGN can be established.

Light microscopy in Type I MPGN reveals a diffuse proliferative glomerulonephritis with an increase in both mesangial cells and matrix.[70, 72, 74] The increase in matrix material often imparts a simplified, lobulated appearance to the glomerular architecture (Fig 5–10,A). The capillary loops and GBM are thickened both by immune-deposits and by the interposition of mesangial cells and matrix between the basement membrane and endothelial cells. Utilizing PAS or silver stains, this matrix has the same tinctoral properties as the

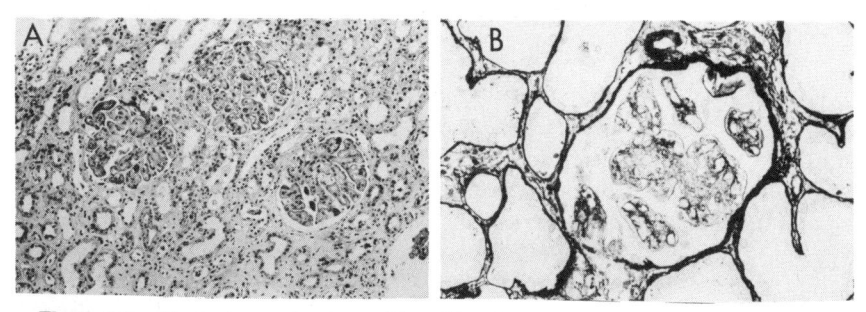

Fig 5–10.—Type I membranoproliferative glomerulonephritis. **A,** hematoxylin-and eosin-stained section demonstrating an increase in both mesangial cells and mesangial matrix and widening of the GBM. The glomeruli exhibit a simplified lobulated appearance. **B,** silver stain of a glomerulus showing the characteristic "splitting" or double contour of the GBM.

original GBM and gives the impression of splitting or duplication of the basement membrane (Fig 5–10,B). Immunofluorescence microscopy discloses immunoglobulins, primarily IgG and IgM, C3, Clq, C4, and properdin along capillary loops and in the mesangium.[70, 74] This pattern has been interpreted to suggest primary activation of the complement system through the classical pathway with subsequent recruitment of the alternative pathway (see below). Ultrastructural examination of renal tissue confirms the light microscopic findings and, in addition, demonstrates subendothelial and mesangial electron-dense deposits.[70, 74] Subepithelial deposits are found in about one third of cases and have led some workers to designate a third type of MPGN. Most investigators, however, consider patients with subepithelial deposits part of the clinical and histologic spectrum of Type I MPGN.[68, 71, 73]

The light microscopic findings are similar in Type I and Type II MPGN; however, the increase in mesangial cells and matrix is usually less prominent in Type II. Glomerular sclerosis and crescent formation have been described occasionally with both varieties of MPGN and predict a relatively rapid progression to ESRD.[68, 75] Immunofluorescence microscopy reveals mesangial and GBM staining for C3, C4, and properdin in Type II MPGN. Immunoglobulins, especially IgG, and Clq are infrequently demonstrated.[70, 71, 74] The characteristic ultrastructural findings in Type II MPGN consist of a ribbon-like, highly electron-dense material deposited along the GBM. Subendothelial and subepithelial deposits are characteristically absent.

Pathophysiology

There are no experimental models of MPGN. Speculation regarding the pathogenesis of MPGN has focused on the striking abnormalities of complement components found in both types of the disorder. Extensive investigation during the past two decades has revealed distinctive patterns of complement abnormalities in each type of MPGN.[68, 74, 76, 77] One third of patients with Type I MPGN have reduced serum concentrations of C3 when the disease is first diagnosed; 50% manifest decreased levels of C3 at some time during their course.[68, 74, 77] Moreover, concentrations of C1q, C4, and properdin are often reduced in Type I disease. C3 nephritic factor (C3Nef), an autoantibody that stabilizes C3 convertase and allows unrestrained alternative pathway activation, is found in 30% of patients with Type I MPGN.[68, 74, 77] Taken together with the immunopathologic findings, these results suggest that Type I MPGN may be an immune-complex disorder mediated, in part, by activation of the classical complement pathway. Recent studies by Coleman et al. support this hypothesis.[78] These investigators found that one quarter of their patients with Type I MPGN had persistent deficiencies of various complement components. By analogy to the immune-complex diseases that occur with increased frequency in patients with inherited deficiencies of complement, they speculated that at least some cases of Type I MPGN might be mediated by immune-complex deposition.

In Type II MPGN, C3 concentrations are reduced at the outset in two thirds and at some time during the disease in 75%.[68, 77] Further, C3 levels are often persistently decreased in contrast to Type I where concentrations often fluctuate. The early components of the classical pathway, C1q and C4, are generally normal.[74, 77] C3Nef is present in most, but not all, patients at some time during the disease. These serologic findings, coupled with the paucity of immunoglobulin deposition in renal tissue, support the notion that activation of the alternative complement pathway is pathogenetically linked to the development of Type II MPGN. Studies in patients with partial lipodystrophy provide further circumstantial evidence.[79, 80] Sissons and colleagues found that 17 of 21 patients with partial lipodystrophy had decreased serum concentrations of C3 and normal levels of C2 and C4; 14 of those 17 had detectable C3Nef.[80] Seven patients had clinically overt glomerulonephritis, and renal biopsy revealed MPGN in six. A few patients with lipodystrophy have Type I disease, but the vast majority manifest both the serologic and histologic characteristics of Type II MPGN. These observations imply that persistent activation of the alternative complement pathway may predispose to the development of Type II MPGN.

Clinical Features

There are few differences in the clinical presentation between Type I and Type II MPGN.[68] Approximately 50% of patients with MPGN have the nephrotic syndrome at the onset of their disease, but 70% eventually develop heavy proteinuria (Table 5–1). Hypertension is present in 40% and over one half have some reduction in GFR at the time of diagnosis. One quarter of subjects present clinically with the acute nephritic syndrome (hypertension, proteinuria, and hematuria) while another 25% have asymptomatic proteinuria or hematuria.[68, 81, 82] Gross or microscopic hematuria are almost invariable features in MPGN and are present in 90% of patients.

Complement profiles differ in Type I and Type II MPGN. Serial determinations of C3 or total hemolytic complement have shown variable hypocomplementemia in Type I disease. As many as 50% of patients exhibit normal C3 levels throughout their course; the remainder often demonstrate fluctuating levels while a few have persistent hypocomplementemia.[68, 70, 74, 81] In contrast, sustained reductions in complement levels are characteristic of Type II MPGN (Fig 5–11).[71]

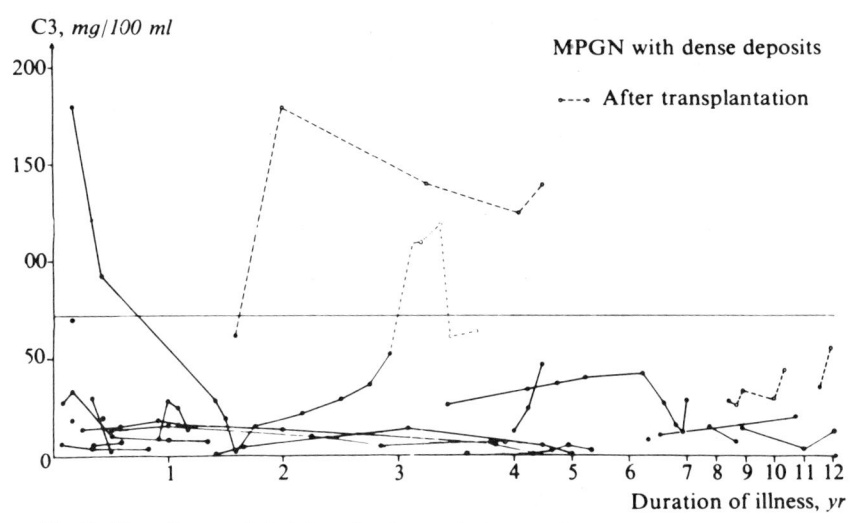

Fig 5–11.—Sequential determinations of plasma C3 concentration in patients with Type II MPGN. (Courtesy of Habib R., et al.: *Kidney Int.* 7:204, 1975.)

Two thirds have persistent hypocomplementemia and over 90% demonstrate decreased concentrations of C3 at some time during their disease.[68, 71, 74] Concentrations of the early acting classical pathway components, Clq and C4, are often low in Type I MPGN but normal in Type II. However, overlap in complement profiles is significant, and isolated determinations or serial measurement of components other than C3 are difficult to interpret. Moreover, even C3 levels correlate poorly with disease activity.

The clinical course of MPGN has been well characterized. Only 5% to 10% of patients undergo spontaneous remission.[68, 74, 83] The vast majority exhibit persistent or intermittent heavy proteinuria, the nephrotic syndrome, or asymptomatic proteinuria and hematuria.[68, 83] Virtually all investigators agree that the prognosis is less favorable in Type II than in Type I MPGN.[68, 70, 71, 74] In both diseases there is usually an inexorable progression to ESRD; however, 50% of patients with Type II disease develop renal failure within 10 years, whereas 17 to 18 years are required before a similar percentage of patients with Type I MPGN reach ESRD.[71, 74] The finding of crescents on renal biopsy predicts a more rapid progression to renal failure irrespective of the type of MPGN.[74, 75]

Therapy

There is no uniformly accepted therapeutic approach to MPGN. The infrequent occurrence of the disease, its indolent course, and the lack of large numbers of controlled, randomized studies do not allow firm conclusions regarding the efficacy of various treatment regimens. Further, since there are few patients with Type II MPGN in any one study, most results are applicable only to Type I disease.

Studies regarding the effect of corticosteroid therapy in MPGN have provided conflicting results. Although there are no prospective, randomized trials of steroid treatment, most investigators suggest that steroid therapy does not beneficially influence the course of the disease.[24, 81] On the other hand, West and co-workers have suggested that long-term alternate day prednisone treatment results in stabilization of both renal function and histology.[72, 84, 85] Because their studies utilized historical controls and excluded a large number of patients, the results must be interpreted with caution. Increased interest in the role of platelets in glomerular disease and the finding of reduced platelet survival in patients with MPGN, have prompted a number of recent investigations examining the effect of antithrombotic therapy in MPGN.[69, 83, 86, 87] Two studies have claimed beneficial effects and one has not been able to demonstrate any difference between the treated and control groups.[69, 86, 87] Given the conflicting results and the potential hazards of long-term steroid or antithrombotic therapy, our policy is to employ only symptomatic treatment in subjects with MPGN (see Chapter 6).

Many patients with MPGN ultimately progress to ESRD and require maintenance dialysis or renal transplantation. Early experience with transplantation in MPGN suggested a high rate of recurrence in the renal allograft.[74, 75, 88, 89] Because chronic allograft rejection can histologically mimic idiopathic Type I MPGN, the 50% recurrence rate in some studies may be an overestimate. Although MPGN, especially Type II disease, can recur in the transplanted kidney, it rarely results in progressive renal dysfunction.[70, 82, 90] Consequently, we do not disallow the use of live, related donors in transplant recipients with MPGN.

MISCELLANEOUS PROLIFERATIVE LESIONS

In 10% or less of all cases, INS results from one of a variety of proliferative glomerulopathies (Table 5–1). For the most part, large series of a single histologic type have not been reported. Two notable exceptions are mesangioproliferative glomerulonephritis and IgA nephropathy. Each has a distinct histologic pattern, well-defined clinical presentation, and characteristic clinical course.[39, 91]

Mesangioproliferative glomerulonephritis accounts for approximately 5% of cases of INS in both children and adults. Age at onset ranges from 2 to 65 with an average age of 25 years. The pathogenesis of mesangioproliferative glomerulonephritis is unknown, but its relationship to both MCD and FGS has engendered much debate (see above). Light microscopy reveals essentially normal glomeruli except for a mild, diffuse increase in mesangial cells and matrix. Immunofluorescence microscopy is often negative but occasionally demonstrates mesangial staining for IgM or C3 or both. Mesangial electron-dense deposits are seen in 25% of cases; effacement of epithelial foot processes is found in over half of the patients with heavy proteinuria.[39]

Approximately one third of patients with mesangioproliferative glomerulonephritis present with the nephrotic syndrome at the onset of their disease; the remainder have either gross or microscopic hematuria or asymptomatic proteinuria as their initial clinical manifestation.[39] The long-term prognosis is excellent, irrespective of the mode of presentation. In general, subjects with mesangioproliferative glomerulonephritis and the nephrotic syndrome respond to corticosteroid and cytotoxic drug therapy in a fashion similar to patients with MCD.[39]

Berger's disease, or IgA nephropathy, is an unusual cause of INS. The disease most commonly affects children and young adults, with peak incidence in the third decade.[91] The pathogenesis of IgA nephropathy is unknown but the temporal relation of upper respiratory or gastrointestinal infections to clinical exacerbations has led most investigators to postulate various immunologic mechanisms. Histologic examination of renal tissue from patients with IgA nephropathy reveals several pathologic lesions. Light microscopy generally demonstrates either diffuse mesangial proliferation, focal segmental glomerulonephritis, or focal sclerosis. The light microscopic findings are usually consistent for an individual case. Mesangial staining for IgA or immunofluorescence microscopy is the pathognomonic finding in IgA nephropathy. Electron microscopy confirms the light microscopic findings and reveals mesangial and paramesangial electron-dense deposits. The majority of patients with IgA nephropathy present with intermittent or persistent, gross or microscopic hematuria.[91] Hypertension is common and renal insufficiency eventually develops in 10% to 20% of cases. Heavy proteinuria is an unusual initial clinical manifestation; the nephrotic syndrome is present in less than 10% of patients at the outset of the disease.[91] Neither corticosteroids nor cytotoxic drug therapy are of proven benefit in IgA nephropathy.

REFERENCES

1. Row P.G., Cameron J.S., Turner D.R., et al.: Membranous nephropathy: Long-term follow-up and association with neoplasia. *Q. J. Med.* 44:207, 1975.
2. Pierides A.M., Malasit P., Morley A.R., et al.: Idiopathic membranous nephropathy. *Q. J. Med.* 46:163, 1977.
3. Arnaout M.A., Rennke H.G., Cotran R.S.: Membranous glomerulonephritis, in Brenner B.M., Stein J.H. (eds.): *Contemporary Issues in Nephrology: Nephrotic Syndrome.* New York, Churchill Livingstone, Inc., 1982, pp. 199–235.
4. Kleinknecht C., Levy M., Gagnadoux M-F., et al.: Membranous glomerulonephritis with extra-renal disorders in children. *Medicine* 58:219, 1979.
5. Ehrenreich T., Porush J.G., Churg J., et al.: Treatment of idiopathic membranous nephropathy. *N. Engl. J. Med.* 295:741, 1976.
6. Cameron J.S.: Pathogenesis and treatment of membranous nephropathy. *Kidney Int.* 15:88, 1979.
7. Franklin W.A., Jennings R.B., Earle D.P.: Membranous glomerulonephritis: long-term serial observations on clinical course and morphology. *Kidney Int.* 4:36, 1973.
8. Zager R.A., Couser W.G., Andrews B.S., et al.: Membranous nephropathy: A radioimmunologic search for anti-renal tubular epithelial antibodies and circulating immune complexes. *Nephron* 24:10, 1979.
9. Ozawa T., Pluss R., Lacher J., et al.: Endogenous immune complex nephropathy

associated with malignancy: I. Studies on the nature and immunopathogenetic significance of glomerular bound antigen and antibody, isolation and characterization of tumor specific antigen and antibody and circulating immune complexes. *Q. J. Med.* 44:523, 1975.
10. Douglas M.F.S., Rabideau D.P., Schwartz M.M., et al.: Evidence of autologous immune-complex nephritis. *N. Engl. J. Med.* 305:1326, 1981.
11. Peters D.K., Lachmann P.J.: Immunity deficiency in pathogenesis of glomerulonephritis. *Lancet* 1:58, 1974.
12. Ooi B.S., Ooi Y.M., Hsu A., et al.: Diminished synthesis of immunoglobulin by peripheral lymphocytes of patients with idiopathic membranous glomerulopathy. *Kidney Int.* 65:789, 1980.
13. Couser W.G., Salant D.J.: In situ immune complex formation and glomerular injury. *Kidney Int.* 17:1, 1980.
14. Cotran R.S., Rennke H.G.: Anionic sites and the mechanisms of proteinuria. *N. Engl. J. Med.* 309:1050, 1983.
15. Couser W.G.: What are circulating immune complexes doing in glomerulonephritis? *N. Engl. J. Med.* 304:1230, 1981.
16. Noel L.H., Zanetti M., Droz D., et al.: Long-term prognosis of idiopathic membranous glomerulonephritis: Study of 116 untreated patients. *Am. J. Med.* 66:82, 1979.
17. Wagoner R.D., Stanson A.W., Holley K.E., et al.: Renal vein thrombosis in idiopathic membranous glomerulopathy and nephrotic syndrome: Incidence and significance. *Kidney Int.* 23:368, 1983.
18. Kauffman R.H., De Graeff J., De La Riviere G.B., et al.: Unilateral renal vein thrombosis and nephrotic syndrome. *Am. J. Med.* 60:1048, 1976.
19. Manos J., Short C.D., Acheson E.J., et al.: Relapsing idiopathic membranous nephropathy. *Clin. Nephrol.* 18:286, 1982.
20. Black D.A.F., Rose G., Brewer D.B.: Controlled trial of prednisone in adult patients with the nephrotic syndrome. *Br. Med. J.* 3:421, 1970.
21. Medical Research Council Working Party: Controlled trial of azathioprin and prednisone in chronic renal disease. *Br. Med. J.* 2:239, 1971.
22. Donadio J.V., Holley K.E., Anderson C.F.: Controlled trial of cyclophosphamide in idiopathic membranous nephropathy. *Kidney Int.* 6:431, 1974.
23. Collaborative Study of the Adult Idiopathic Nephrotic Syndrome: A controlled study of short-term prednisone treatment in adults with membranous nephropathy. *N. Engl. J. Med.* 310:1301, 1979.
24. Relman A.S.: Steroids to prevent uremia. *N. Engl. J. Med.* 301:1340, 1979.
25. Ponticelli C., Zucchelli P., Imbasciati E., et al.: Controlled trial of methylprednisolone and chlorambucil in idiopathic membranous glomerulopathy. *N. Engl. J. Med.* 310:946, 1984.
26. Lim V.S., Sibley R., Spargo B.H.: Adult lipoid nephrosis: clinicopathologic correlations. *Ann. Intern. Med.* 81:314, 1974.
27. Hoyer J.R.: Idiopathic nephrotic syndrome with minimal glomerular changes, in Brenner B.M., Stein J.H. (eds.): *Contemporary Issues in Nephrology: Nephrotic Syndrome*. New York, Churchill Livingstone, Inc., 1982, pp. 145–174.
28. Siegel N.J., Gaudio K.M., Krassner L.S., et al.: Steroid-dependent nephrotic syndrome in children: Histopathology and relapses after cyclophosphamide treatment. *Kidney Int.* 19:454, 1981.
29. Levinsky R.J., Malleson P.N., Barratt T.M., et al.: Circulating immune complexes in steroid-responsive nephrotic syndrome. *N. Engl. J. Med.* 298:135, 1978.
30. Meltzer J.I., Keim H.J., Laragh J.H., et al.: Nephrotic syndrome: vasoconstriction and hypervolemic types indicated by renin-sodium profiling. *Ann. Intern. Med.* 91:688, 1979.
31. Pru C., Kjellstrand C.M., Cohu R.A., et al.: Late recurrence of minimal lesion nephrotic syndrome. *Ann. Intern. Med.* 100:69, 1984.

32. Raij L., Keane W.F., Leonard A., et al.: Irreversible acute renal failure in idiopathic nephrotic syndrome. *Am. J. Med.* 61:207, 1976.
33. Lowenstein J., Schacht R.G., Baldwin D.S.: Renal failure in minimal change nephrotic syndrome. *Am. J. Med.* 70:227, 1981.
34. Arbeitsgemeinschaft fur Padiatrische Nephrologie: Effect of cytotoxic drugs in frequently relapsing nephrotic syndrome with and without steroid dependence. *N. Engl. J. Med.* 306:451, 1982.
35. International Study of Kidney Disease in Children: Prospective, controlled trial of cyclophosphamide therapy in children with the nephrotic syndrome. *Lancet* 2:423, 1974.
36. Williams S.A., Makker S.P., Ingelfinger J.R., et al.: Long-term evaluation of chlorambucil plus prednisone in the idiopathic nephrotic syndrome of childhood. *N. Engl. J. Med.* 302:929, 1980.
37. Southwest Pediatric Nephrology Study Group: Childhood nephrotic syndrome associated with diffuse mesangial hypercellularity. *Kidney Int.* 23:867, 1983.
38. Jao W., Pollack V.E., Norris S.H., et al.: Lipoid nephrosis: an approach to the clinicopathologic analysis and dismemberment of idiopathic nephrotic syndrome with minimal glomerular changes. *Medicine* 58:295, 1979.
39. Brown E.A., Upadhyaya K., Hayslett J.P., et al.: The clinical course of mesangial proliferative glomerulonephritis. *Medicine* 58:295, 1979.
40. Shalhoub R.J.: Pathogenesis of lipoid nephrosis: A disorder of T-cell function. *Lancet* 2:556, 1974.
41. Couser W., Badger A., Cooperband S., et al.: Hodgkin's disease and lipoid nephrosis. *Lancet* 1:912, 1977.
42. Giangiacomo J., Cleary T.G., Cole B.R.: Serum immunoglobulins in the nephrotic syndrome: A possible cause of minimal-change nephrotic syndrome. *N. Engl. J. Med.* 293:6, 1975.
43. Nagata K., Platt J.L., Michael A.F.: Interstitial and glomerular immune cell populations in idiopathic nephrotic syndrome. *Kidney Int.* 25:88, 1984.
44. Trompeter R.S., Barratt T.M., Kay R., et al.: HLA, atopy and cyclophosphamide in steroid-responsive childhood nephrotic syndrome. *Kidney Int.* 17:113, 1980.
45. Carrie B., Salyer W.R., Myers B.D.: Minimal change nephropathy: an electrochemical disorder of the glomerular membrane. *Am. J. Med.* 70:262, 1981.
46. Bridges C.R., Myers B.D., Brenner B.M., et al.: Glomerular charge alterations in human minimal change nephropathy. *Kidney Int.* 22:677, 1982.
47. Mees E.J., Roos J.C., Boer P., et al.: Observations on edema formation in the nephrotic syndrome in adults with minimal lesions. *Am. J. Med.* 67:378, 1979.
48. Hulter H.N., Bonner E.L.: Lipoid nephrosis appearing as acute oliguric renal failure. *Arch. Intern. Med.* 140:403, 1980.
49. Hopper J., Ryan P., Lee J.C., et al.: Lipoid nephrosis in 31 adult patients: Renal biopsy by light, electron and fluorescent microscopy with experience in treatment. *Medicine* 49:321, 1970.
50. Idelson B.A., Smithline N., Smith G.W., et al.: Prognosis in steroid treated idiopathic nephrotic syndrome in adults. *Arch. Intern. Med.* 137:891, 1977.
51. Lewis E.J.: Chlorambucil for childhood nephrosis. *N. Engl. J. Med.* 302:963, 1980.
52. Feehally J., Beattie T.J., Brenchly P.E.C., et al.: Modulation of cellular immune function by cyclophosphamide in children with minimal change nephropathy. *N. Engl. J. Med.* 310:415, 1984.
53. Kida H., Kida H., Dohi K., et al.: Period of freedom from relapse as an indication of cure in minimal change nephrotic syndrome in adults. *Nephron* 19:153, 1977.
54. Goldszer R.C., Sweet J., Cotran R.S.: Focal segmental glomerulosclerosis. *Annu. Rev. Med.* 35:429, 1984.
55. Tisher C.C., Alexander R.W.: Focal glomerular sclerosis, in Brenner B., Stein J.H. (eds.): *Contemporary Issues in Nephrology: Nephrotic Syndrome.* New York, Churchill Livingstone, Inc., 1982, pp. 175–197.

56. Jenis E.W., Teichmann S., Briggs W.A., et al.: Focal segmental glomerulosclerosis. *Am. J. Med.* 57:695, 1974.
57. Newman W.J., Tisher C.C., McCoy R.C., et al.: Focal glomerular sclerosis: Contrasting clinical patterns in children and adults: *Medicine* 55:67, 1976.
58. Velosa J.A., Donadio J.V., Holley K.D.: Focal sclerosing glomerulopathy: A clinicopathologic study. *Mayo Clin. Proc.* 50:121, 1975.
59. Saint-Hillier Y., Morel-Maroger L., Woodrow D., et al.: Focal and segmental hyalinosis. *Adv. Nephrol.* 5:67, 1975.
60. Matalon R., Katz L., Gallo G., et al.: Glomerular sclerosis in adults with nephrotic syndrome. *Ann. Intern. Med.* 80:488, 1974.
61. Rich A.R.: A hitherto undescribed vulnerability of the juxtamedullary glomeruli in lipid nephrosis. *Bull. J. Hopkins Hosp.* 100:173, 1957.
62. Taylor J., Novak R., Christiansen R., et al.: Focal sclerosing glomerulopathy with adverse effects during pregnancy. *Arch. Intern. Med.* 138:1695, 1978.
63. Southwest Pediatric Nephrology Study Group: Focal segmental glomerulosclerosis in children with idiopathic nephrotic syndrome. A report of the Southwest Pediatric Nephrology Study Group. *Kidney Int.* 27:442, 1985.
64. Geary D.F., Farine M., Thorner P., et al.: Response to cyclophosphamide in steroid-resistant focal segmental glomerulosclerosis: A reappraisal. *Clin. Nephrol.* 22:109, 1984.
65. Maizel S.E., Sibley R.K., Horstinan J.P., et al.: Incidence and significance of recurrent focal segmental glomerulosclerosis in renal allograft recipients. *Transplantation* 32:512, 1981.
66. Lewis E.J.: Recurrent focal sclerosis after renal transplantation. *Kidney Int.* 22:315, 1982.
67. Torres V.E., Velosa J.A., Holley K.E., et al.: Meclofenamate treatment of recurrent idiopathic nephrotic syndrome with focal segmental glomerulosclerosis after renal transplantation. *Mayo Clin. Proc.* 59:146, 1984.
68. Cameron J.S., Turner D.R., Heaton J., et al.: Idiopathic mesangiocapillary glomerulonephritis: Comparison of Types I and II in children and adults and long-term prognosis. *Am. J. Med.* 74:175, 1983.
69. Cattran D.C., Cardella C.J., Roscoe J.M., et al.: Results of a controlled drug trial in membranoproliferative glomerulonephritis. *Kidney Int.* 27:436, 1985.
70. Kim Y., Michael A.F., Fish A.J.: Idiopathic membranoproliferative glomerulonephritis, in Brenner B.M., Stein J.H. (eds.): *Contemporary Issues in Nephrology: Nephrotic Syndrome.* New York, Churchill Livingstone, Inc., 1982, pp. 237–257.
71. Habib R., Gubler M-C., Loirat C., et al.: Dense deposit disease: A variant of membranoproliferative glomerulonephritis. *Kidney Int.* 7:204, 1975.
72. West C.D.: Pathogenesis and approaches to therapy of membranoproliferative glomerulonephritis. *Kidney Int.* 9:1, 1976.
73. Case Records of the M.G.H.: *N. Engl. J. Med.* 307:1000, 1982.
74. Kim Y., Michael A.F.: Idiopathic membranoproliferative glomerulonephritis. *Annu. Rev. Med.* 31:273, 1980.
75. McCoy R.C., Clapp J., Seigler H.F.: Membranoproliferative glomerulonephritis: Progression from the pure form to the crescentic form with recurrence after transplantation. *Am. J. Med.* 59:288, 1975.
76. Fearon D.T.: Glomerulonephritis, complement and C3NeF. *N. Engl. J. Med.* 294:495, 1976.
77. Ooi Y.M., Vallota E.H., West C.D.: Classical complement pathway activation in membranoproliferative glomerulonephritis. *Kidney Int.* 9:46, 1976.
78. Coleman T.H., Forristal J., Kosaka T., et al.: Inherited complement component deficiencies in membranoproliferative glomerulonephritis. *Kidney Int.* 24:681, 1983.
79. Peters D.K., Charlesworth J.A., Sissons J.G.P., et al.: Mesangiocapillary nephritis, partial lipodystrophy and hypocomplementemia. *Lancet* 2:535, 1973.

80. Sissons J.G.P., West R.J., Fallows J., et al.: The complement abnormalities of lipodystrophy. *N. Engl. J. Med.* 294:461, 1976.
81. Cameron J.S., Glasgow E.F., Ogg C.S.: Membranoproliferative glomerulonephritis and persistent hypocomplementemia. *Br. Med. J.* 4:7, 1970.
82. Sibley R.K., Kim Y.: Dense intramembranous deposit disease: new pathologic features. *Kidney Int.* 25:660, 1984.
83. Hayslett J.P.: Role of platelets in glomerulonephritis. *N. Engl. J. Med.* 310:1457, 1984.
84. McAdams A.J., McEnry P.T., West C.D.: Mesangiocapillary glomerulonephritis: Changes in glomerular morphology with long-term alternate day prednisone therapy. *Pediatrics* 86:23, 1975.
85. McEnery P.T., McAdams A.J., West C.D.: Membranoproliferative glomerulonephritis: Improved survival with alternate day prednisone therapy. *Clin. Nephrol.* 13:117, 1980.
86. Zimmerman S.W., Moorthy A.V., Dreher W.H., et al.: Prospective trial of warfarin and dipyridamole in patients with membranoproliferative glomerulonephritis. *Am. J. Med.* 75:920, 1983.
87. Donadio J.V., Anderson C.F., Mitchell J.C., et al.: Membranoproliferative glomerulonephritis: A prospective clinical trial of platelet-inhibitor therapy. *N. Engl. J. Med.* 310:1421, 1984.
88. Zimmerman S.W., Hyman L.R., Uehling D.T., et al.: Recurrent membranoproliferative glomerulonephritis with glomerular properdin deposition in allografts. *Ann. Intern. Med.* 80:169, 1974.
89. McLean R.H., Geiger H., Burke B., et al.: Recurrence of membranoproliferative glomerulonephritis following kidney transplantation. *Am. J. Med.* 60:60, 1976.
90. Curtis J.J., Wyatt R.J., Bhathena D., et al.: Renal transplantation for patients with Type I and Type II membranoproliferative glomerulonephritis. *Am. J. Med.* 66:216, 1979.
91. Kincaid-Smith P., Nicholls K.: Mesangial IgA nephropathy. *Am. J. Kid. Dis.* 3:90, 1983.

6 *Diagnosis and General Management of the Proteinuric Patient*

MANAGEMENT OF THE PATIENT with proteinuria begins with the recognition of qualitative and quantitative patterns of urinary protein excretion outlined in Chapter 1. Specific therapies for disorders associated with heavy proteinuria and the nephrotic syndrome are discussed in Chapters 4 and 5. In this chapter, we review the general management of patients with proteinuria. We first discuss the clinical assessment and management of patients with intermittent or asymptomatic proteinuria. We then review the initial clinical assessment of patients with the nephrotic syndrome, explore the role of renal biopsy, and discuss the treatment of metabolic abnormalities associated with heavy proteinuria. Because management of children with nephrotic syndrome differs greatly from that of adults, we include a brief discussion of the assessment and management of nephrotic syndrome in children.

Once proteinuria has been documented, patient evaluation begins with a complete history and physical examination focusing on historical features, signs, and symptoms of systemic diseases that can affect the kidney. A family history may reveal evidence of a hereditary renal disease such as Alport's syndrome. A complete list of the patient's medications should be obtained to exclude drug-induced renal disease. Documentation of normal findings on previous urinalyses may allow the physician to accurately date the onset of proteinuria. The physical examination should focus on the presence or absence of edema and hypertension. Initial laboratory evaluation of the proteinuric patient should include measurement of the BUN and serum creatinine concentration (as estimates of glomerular filtration rate) and a careful urinalysis (including examination of the sediment of a freshly voided specimen). Quantitation of urinary protein in a 24-

ASSESSMENT AND MANAGEMENT OF PATIENTS WITH INTERMITTENT OR ASYMPTOMATIC PROTEINURIA

By definition, patients with intermittent or asymptomatic proteinuria excrete less than 3.0 gm of urinary protein per day, exhibit no signs or symptoms of systemic disease, and have normal renal function without hypertension or renal insufficiency. Patients in this category should be tested for true postural proteinuria (see Chapter 1) since its discovery implies a favorable prognosis and influences the extent and frequency of follow-up examination. The recommended follow-up evaluation for patients with intermittent or asymptomatic proteinuria is summarized in Table 6–1 and discussed below.

Benign Transient Proteinuria

Patients in whom a single positive test for urinary protein cannot be corroborated on subsequent evaluation virtually never have serious underlying renal disease. Because no harmful sequelae have been described in these patients, long-term follow-up is not necessary.

Functional Proteinuria

Functional proteinuria rarely accounts for the excretion of more than 1 to 2 gm of urinary protein per day. Protein excretion of this magnitude has few clinical consequences. Furthermore, urinary protein excretion typically returns to normal after recovery from the pre-

TABLE 6–1.—RECOMMENDED FOLLOW-UP EVALUATION OF PATIENTS WITH INTERMITTENT OR ASYMPTOMATIC PROTEINURIA*

PATTERN OF PROTEINURIA	RISK OF CHRONIC RENAL FAILURE	RECOMMENDED EVALUATION	INVERVAL (YEARS)
Transient	None	None	—
Functional	None	None	—
Postural	Very slight, if any	Blood pressure, urinalysis, postural protein analysis	1–2
Persistent, asymptomatic	20% after 10 years	Blood pressure, urinalysis, BUN serum creatinine	0.5–1.0

*Modified from Abuelo.[4]

cipitating disorder. Investigation for underlying renal disease should be pursued only if proteinuria persists after resolution of the underlying disorder (see Chapter 1).

Postural Proteinuria

Patients with true postural proteinuria appear to have a very low risk for developing progressive renal disease; however, follow-up studies of patients with a postural pattern of proteinuria have yielded conflicting results regarding the natural history of this disorder. While some studies suggest that a large fraction of patients with postural proteinuria develop persistent proteinuria,[1] others indicate that postural proteinuria slowly remits with time.[2,3] Until the long-term consequences of postural proteinuria are more precisely defined, it is prudent to evaluate such patients every one to two years as long as proteinuria persists.[4] In addition to monitoring the patient's blood pressure and urinalysis during these infrequent visits, supine and upright urine collections should be analyzed to exclude the development of persistent proteinuria or to document remission (see Chapter 1). Although minor histologic abnormalities are found in as many as half of patients with postural proteinuria,[5] renal biopsy has little value in the routine management of these patients since specific therapy is not warranted.

Persistent Asymptomatic Proteinuria

Persistent proteinuria almost invariably reflects renal parenchymal injury even when the patient has no signs or symptoms of renal disease, when the urine sediment contains no abnormalities, and when glomerular filtration rate is normal. Because the risk for developing hypertension and renal insufficiency is greater among patients with persistent asymptomatic proteinuria than in individuals without proteinuria (see Chapter 1), patients with this pattern of protein excretion should be evaluated once or twice yearly for blood pressure measurement, urinalysis, and determination of renal function by measurement of the BUN and serum creatinine concentration.[4]

Intravenous pyelography and/or renal ultrasonography should be obtained during the evaluation of patients with asymptomatic proteinuria since this pattern of proteinuria is occasionally associated with obstructive uropathies,[6] chronic interstitial nephritis, or vesicoureteral reflux.[7] Diabetes mellitus should be excluded in all patients with otherwise unexplained proteinuria, regardless of the magnitude of urinary protein excretion. Other laboratory studies must be individualized. Serum and urine protein electrophoreses are reasonable screening tests in older patients in whom asymptomatic proteinuria may be the first sign of a monoclonal gammopathy. Extensive serologic studies such as serum complement levels and antinuclear antibodies are not warranted in the routine assessment of patients with asymptomatic proteinuria. Although the detection of hypocomplementemia is invaluable in the differential diagnosis of glomerular diseases, its discovery rarely influences the management of the patient with asymptomatic proteinuria.

Approximately 20% of patients with asymptomatic proteinuria have readily identifiable glomerular lesions.[4] The remaining patients may have mild mesangioproliferative changes, tubulointerstitial disease, or normal histologic findings. Renal biopsy can be performed to determine the precise pathology, but rarely provides data of therapeutic value in this category of proteinuric patients. Thus, renal biopsy is rarely warranted in the routine management of patients with asymptomatic proteinuria.

No specific therapy can be recommended for patients with persistent asymptomatic proteinuria because few controlled clinical studies have explored the role of corticosteroids, cytotoxic agents, or other drugs in this group of patients. As mentioned above, blood pressure should be monitored closely and hypertension treated aggressively, especially in patients with established renal insufficiency. The latter recommendation is based on the presumption that control of hypertension may retard the rate of progression of the underlying renal disease—a phenomenon that has been clearly demonstrated in patients with diabetic nephropathy.[8,9]

ASSESSMENT AND MANAGEMENT OF PATIENTS WITH HEAVY PROTEINURIA AND THE NEPHROTIC SYNDROME

Clinical and Laboratory Assessment of Patients with the Nephrotic Syndrome

The initial task of the physician evaluating the patient with nephrotic syndrome is to ascertain whether the disorder is primary (idiopathic) or secondary to systemic illness. Because the clinical features of primary and secondary nephrotic syndrome often overlap, the physician is obliged to consider secondary forms of the disorder in all patients presenting with heavy proteinuria. Diagnostic investigation of the nephrotic patient begins with a careful history and physical examination. In addition to providing evidence for the presence or absence of systemic disorders associated with secondary nephrotic syndrome, the initial examination allows the physician to assess the patient's overall nutritional status as well as the degree and severity of edema, hypertension, or hypotension—parameters that greatly influence general management of the nephrotic patient.

Given the diverse causes of secondary nephrotic syndrome, the extent of the diagnostic investigation to assess the presence or absence of various diseases must be individualized, keeping in mind certain epidemiologic considerations. For example, secondary nephrotic syndrome is relatively uncommon in the pediatric population in which idiopathic minimal change disease accounts for more than 70% of cases. In the United States, diabetic glomerulosclerosis is the most common cause of secondary nephrotic syndrome in adults and should be considered the most likely diagnosis in patients with longstanding diabetes mellitus. Infectious diseases such as quartan malaria, schistosomiasis, and leprosy predominate as causes of the nephrotic syndrome in other areas of the world. In Japan, membranous glomerulopathy is more commonly associated with hepatitis B antigenemia than in other countries.[10] Heroin nephropathy is most prevalent in urban centers with large populations of drug addicts.[11, 12] Beyond these simple considerations, the physician must be familiar with the natural histories of the more common causes of secondary nephrotic syndrome discussed in Chapter 4.

The medical history and physical examination may provide obvious clues to the presence of a secondary form of nephrotic syndrome. A complete drug and family history may elicit evidence for drug-induced or hereditary renal disease. Sickle cell nephropathy is the likely diagnosis in black patients with sickle cell disease and otherwise unexplained nephrotic syndrome.[13] Fatigue, objective muscle weakness, unexplained cardiac failure, and hepatosplenomegaly are signs and symptoms suggesting amyloidosis. A history of persisting chronic infections such as tuberculosis or osteomyelitis raises suspicion of secondary amyloidosis. Varying combinations of arthralgias, skin rash, fever, pleuropericardial pain, and Raynaud's phenomenon suggest an underlying connective tissue disease such as systemic lupus erythematosus. Purpuric skin lesions associated with nephrotic syndrome suggest systemic vasculitis, essential mixed cryoglobulinemia, or Henoch-Schönlein disease. In patients with longstanding diabetes mellitus and nephrotic syndrome, the concomitant findings of diabetic retinopathy and peripheral neuropathy strongly suggest diabetic glomerulosclerosis as the underlying cause of heavy proteinuria.

Regardless of the cause of nephrotic syndrome, initial laboratory evaluation should include a complete urinalysis, measurement of the serum creatinine concentration, measurement of the serum albumin concentration, and quantitation of urinary protein in a 24-hour urine specimen. The latter two laboratory tests serve to corroborate the diagnosis and provide a preliminary assessment of the severity of the glomerular protein leak as well as a baseline for monitoring the effects of specific therapy. Measurement of serum lipid levels (i.e., serum cholesterol and triglycerides and/or lipoprotein electrophoresis) is probably warranted in the initial laboratory evaluation of all nephrotic patients to verify the diagnosis of nephrotic syndrome and to identify the rare, severely hyperlipidemic patient who may require therapy to reduce serum lipids. Measurement of serum lipids is helpful in evaluation of the nephrotic patient with hyponatremia because severe hyperlipidemia may be associated with spurious or "pseudohyponatremia." In general, the presence and severity of hyperlipidemia and lipiduria in nephrotic syndrome have little diagnostic significance; however, sporadic reports suggest that the absence of hypercholesterolemia in patients with heavy proteinuria favors a diagnosis of proliferative glomerulonephritis or lupus nephritis rather than minimal change disease.[14, 15]

As discussed in Chapter 2, some correlation exists between the selectivity of urinary protein excretion and the underlying glomerular histopathology. A highly selective pattern of proteinuria supports a diagnosis of minimal change disease; however, a poorly selective pattern does not exclude the latter entity and fails to discriminate among a number of other glomerulopathies associated with nephrotic syndrome. Although measurement of a selectivity index is sometimes valuable in the assessment and management of nephrotic children in whom minimal change nephropathy is the most common glomerular lesion, it has proved to be insufficiently discriminating as a diagnostic tool in the evaluation of nephrotic adults.[16] The low risk of renal biopsy relative to its diagnostic yield has made measurement of selectivity less preferable to biopsy as a diagnostic procedure.

Beyond the initial laboratory studies designed to corroborate the diagnosis of nephrotic syndrome and to assess its severity, measurements of fasting blood sugar, total hemolytic complement, and antinuclear antibodies are reasonable screening tests for systemic disease even when the history and physical examination fail to suggest one.

More sophisticated laboratory tests are performed only when the clinical suspicion of a given disease is high. For example, rectal biopsy or subcutaneous fat pad aspiration may be an appropriate test in elderly patients or in those with chronic inflammatory disorders, clinical settings associated with increased frequency of systemic amyloidosis.

As discussed in Chapter 4, a number of studies suggest a higher than chance association of nephrotic syndrome with various malignancies.[17, 18] Hodgkin's disease is particularly associated with minimal change nephropathy, while membranous glomerulopathy is more frequently seen with carcinomas.[19] Should all adults with otherwise unexplained nephrotic syndrome undergo extensive investigation to exclude occult malignancy? Cost-benefit analyses have not been performed to answer this question. Our preference is to seek evidence of a malignancy only when the history, physical examination, and "routine" laboratory studies suggest a neoplastic disease. In membranous glomerulopathy, the most commonly associated tumors are those of the lung, breast, and gastrointestinal tract.[19, 20] Therefore, "routine" studies should include (as a minimum) a chest x-ray, a thorough breast examination, and examination of the stool for occult blood. More extensive studies may be warranted in elderly nephrotic patients with weight loss or other signs suggesting an occult malignancy, especially if the underlying histology is membranous glomerulopathy.

The clinical and laboratory assessment outlined above neither precludes nor replaces the use of renal biopsy in evaluation of patients with the nephrotic syndrome. Renal biopsy is rarely helpful in discriminating primary and secondary nephrotic syndrome because the renal histologic changes associated with secondary forms of nephrotic syndrome often are identical to those seen in the idiopathic varieties (Table 6-2). Thus, the diagnosis of idiopathic nephrotic syndrome is most often a diagnosis of exclusion made on clinical grounds after careful consideration is given to various secondary forms of the disorder.

THE ROLE OF RENAL BIOPSY IN PATIENTS WITH IDIOPATHIC NEPHROTIC SYNDROME

Percutaneous renal biopsy has been employed in the evaluation of patients with renal disease for more than 30 years.[21, 22] The development and routine use of light, immunofluorescence, and electron microscopy in the evaluation of renal biopsy tissue has led to a quantum

TABLE 6–2.—DISORDERS IN WHICH RENAL HISTOPATHOLOGY RESEMBLES
IDIOPATHIC NEPHROTIC SYNDROME

RENAL HISTOPATHOLOGY	DISORDER
Minimal change nephropathy	Hodgkin's disease Lymphoma Bee stings, pollen allergies Drugs—lithium, nonsteroidal anti-inflammatory drugs
Focal glomerulosclerosis	Heroin abuse Allograft rejection Vesicoureteral reflux Analgesic abuse nephropathy
Membranous glomerulopathy	Systemic lupus erythematosus Carcinoma Hepatitis B, malaria, syphilis Drugs—gold, mercurials, penicillamine, captopril
Membranoproliferative glomerulonephritis	Hepatitis B Systemic lupus erythematosus Sjögren's syndrome Cryoglobulinemia Schistosomiasis Sickle cell nephropathy

change in our knowledge of renal disease, giving great impetus for the development of nephrology as a subspecialty.[23] Morbidity and mortality associated with renal biopsy have been reduced greatly by proper patient selection and by the use of sophisticated imaging techniques including fluoroscopy, ultrasonography, and computerized axial tomography. Nevertheless, it has been estimated that important complications, largely related to bleeding, occur in 5% to 10% of cases.[23] Hospitalization is required to prepare the patient for the biopsy and to monitor for serious bleeding immediately following the procedure. Death is a rare, but probably underreported, complication of renal biopsy. Clearly, the cost and risk of renal biopsy must be weighed against its potential benefit when selecting patients for this diagnostic procedure.

Most physicians regard the idiopathic nephrotic syndrome in an adult to be a very strong indication for renal biopsy. As discussed in Chapter 5, the principal glomerular lesions found in patients with idiopathic nephrotic syndrome are: membranous glomerulopathy, minimal change nephropathy, focal glomerulosclerosis, and membranoproliferative glomerulonephritis. Clinical features of these various forms of idiopathic nephrotic syndrome overlap sufficiently so that the histologic lesion cannot be predicted reliably from clinical criteria alone. Renal biopsy is the only highly specific method for determining which glomerular lesion is present. Because the natural history, prognosis, and response to treatment differ among glomerulopathies, identification of the precise histopathology is considered by most nephrologists essential to optimal therapeutic decision making.

The traditional biopsy-directed approach to the management of patients with idiopathic nephrotic syndrome has been a subject of increasing controversy. Because the risk of corticosteroids as they are currently used in the treatment of nephrotic syndrome is low, and especially because steroids are the only therapy with proved efficacy in idiopathic nephrotic syndrome, an alternative strategy might consist of empirically treating all patients with steroids, avoiding the cost and small risk of renal biopsy. Using this approach, biopsy could be reserved for those patients who fail to respond to steroid therapy or for whom an early estimate of prognosis is deemed essential. Decision analysis has been employed to compare the biopsy-directed approach to "blind" treatment with steroids.[24, 25] Even when the risks of renal biopsy and steroid therapy are grossly exaggerated, the expected utilities for the two approaches are virtually identical, so that the choice between these two strategies appears at best to be a "toss-up."[25] It is too early to judge the impact of these preliminary decision analyses on the practice of nephrologists. We suspect that such studies have lowered the threshold of the nephrologic community to prescribe empirical treatment with steroids for patients with idiopathic nephrotic syndrome, especially when renal biopsy is relatively or absolutely contraindicated. Nevertheless, renal biopsy remains an essential tool in research studies investigating the effect of new treatment regimens on the natural history of glomerulopathies associated with nephrotic syndrome.

MANAGEMENT OF METABOLIC ABNORMALITIES ASSOCIATED WITH THE NEPHROTIC SYNDROME

Short of inducing complete remission from proteinuria with specific therapy, management of patients with the nephrotic syndrome entails supportive treatment of the expected consequences and complications of heavy proteinuria. Many of the glomerular diseases underlying the nephrotic syndrome respond poorly to specific therapy, so that patients may remain nephrotic for long periods of time. Thus, the physician caring for the nephrotic patient must be familiar with the principles of supportive management outlined below.

Management of Edema and Hypoalbuminemia

Edema is the most common and most troublesome symptom associated with the nephrotic syndrome. The pathophysiology of edema formation in the nephrotic syndrome is not completely understood (see Chapter 3); however, the severity of edema generally correlates with the magnitude of hypoalbuminemia, and ranges from mild symmetrical ankle swelling to anasarca accompanied by ascites and pleural effusions. Many patients complain of periorbital puffiness that is most prominent on waking in the morning, gradually subsiding during the day as excess interstitial fluid gravitates to more dependent parts of the body. Male patients may note penile and scrotal swelling. Overt pulmonary edema is unusual in the absence of associated heart disease. In patients with severe edema, the skin may spontaneously fissure, predisposing to consequent cellulitis. Because the skin of edematous patients heals slowly following injury, cellulitis may spread very rapidly if not recognized and treated early.

A number of therapeutic maneuvers are available for the management of nephrotic edema. In general, such measures should be employed only when edema produces discomfort or when breakdown of the skin is imminent. Thoracentesis and abdominal paracentesis are occasionally required in the emergent management of patients with pleural effusions or ascites accompanied by respiratory embarrassment. Other therapeutic measures are designed either to counteract secondary renal sodium retention or to alleviate the hypoalbuminemia characteristic of the nephrotic syndrome.

Diet

Unless glomerular filtration rate is significantly impaired, a high protein diet should be prescribed to offset urinary and catabolic protein losses and to provide maximal substrate for hepatic albumin synthesis. In adults, the diet should contain 1.5 to 3 gm of protein per kilogram of body weight. Protein intake in excess of this amount is of no proven therapeutic value. Indeed, a high protein intake may increase the serum albumin concentration and increase the magnitude of proteinuria,[26] suggesting that amino acid availability is self-limiting in the correction of hypoalbuminemia in nephrotic syndrome. Proteins of high biologic value (eggs, milk, meat) should be used to supply 75% of the total protein in the diet.[27]

Dietary restriction of sodium is necessary only for patients with hypertension or symptomatic edema. With the relatively recent development of potent diuretic drugs, too little attention has been paid to the role of dietary sodium restriction in the management of nephrotic edema. Because sodium balance reflects the algebraic sum of dietary intake and urinary excretion of sodium, the institution of a low sodium diet may slow or prevent the accumulation of sodium and water in nephrotic subjects. Diets containing less than 20 mEq of sodium per day can be prescribed for hospitalized patients in whom aggressive diuresis is necessary. Few patients are able to tolerate such severe dietary sodium restriction for long periods. Most adults find a daily dietary sodium allowance of 90 mEq (2 grams) palatable and effective in the control of edema.

Diuretics

A wide variety of diuretic agents is available for the management of edematous disorders (Fig 6–1). In patients with nephrotic syndrome, diuretics are employed to induce negative sodium balance, but these agents must be used judiciously to avoid precipitous reductions

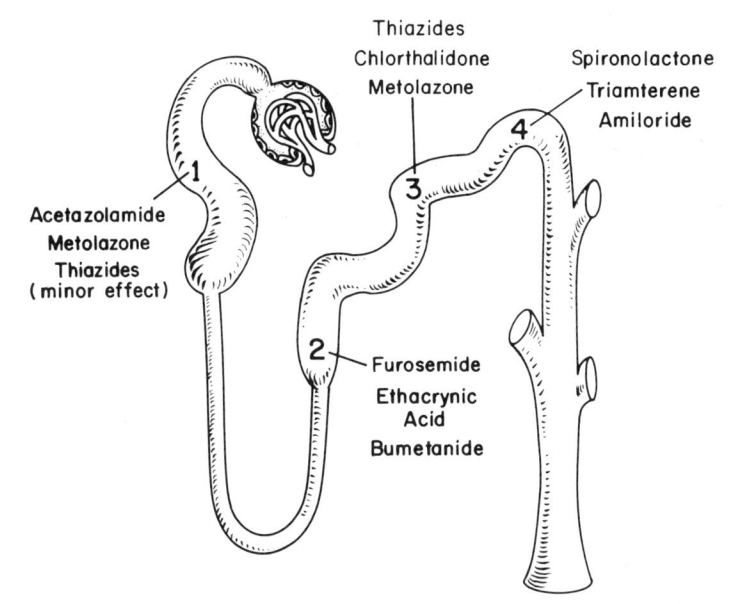

Fig 6–1.—Sites of action of commonly used diuretics. *1*, proximal tubule. *2*, thick ascending limb of Henle's loop. *3*, early distal tubule. *4*, late distal tubule.

in intravascular volume. Given the dangers of diuretic-induced plasma volume depletion, these drugs should be prescribed only for patients with symptomatic edema that cannot be controlled with dietary sodium restriction alone.

When treating outpatients, a small dose of a thiazide diuretic or furosemide should be prescribed to initiate therapy. Patients should be instructed to weigh themselves daily and to discontinue the diuretic if weight loss amounts to more than 2 to 3 pounds per day. It is also important to instruct the patient to reduce or eliminate the diuretic when a small amount of edema remains. Hospitalization may be required to monitor diuresis in patients with severe edema and profound hypoalbuminemia. In addition to following the patient closely for clinical signs of intravascular volume depletion, the BUN and serum creatinine concentration should be monitored for signs of prerenal azotemia that warrant a reduction in the dose of the diuretic.

Patients with nephrotic syndrome not infrequently exhibit resistance to the natriuretic effect of single diuretic drugs. Diuretic "resistance" in this setting may simply reflect inadequate dietary sodium restriction or poor absorption of orally administered drugs consequent to edema of the intestinal wall. True resistance to a diuretic agent usually indicates compensatory sodium absorption at nephronal sites other than the transport site sensitive to the specific drug. For example, the thiazides and "loop" diuretics (furosemide, ethacrynic acid, bumetanide) each block sodium chloride absorption at tubular sites proximal to the aldosterone-sensitive portions of the distal tubule. Because many nephrotic patients exhibit intense secondary hyperaldosteronism, a large portion of the sodium chloride remaining in the tubular lumen may be recaptured by the more distal sites where sodium is absorbed in exchange for potassium and hydrogen ions under the influence of aldosterone. In addition, proximal tubular sodium absorption may be increased in the presence of a distally acting diuretic drug.[28] Resistance to therapy with a single diuretic agent is managed by increasing the dose of the drug or by prescribing a combination of diuretics that block sodium reabsorption at different tubular sites. In our experience, it is rarely beneficial to increase the dose of furosemide above 500 mg per day. The addition of spironolactone, triamterene, or amiloride may effectively block distal sites of sodium absorption, and is particularly advantageous in the management of patients with diuretic-induced hypokalemia. These "potassium-sparing" diuretics should be used with great caution in patients with diabetes mellitus and should be avoided in patients with renal functional impairment. The addition of thiazides or metolazone to furosemide is a very potent diuretic combination and may be required by a few patients who are refractory to loop diuretics alone. This combination can cause severe volume depletion and should be used with careful monitoring of the patient's volume status.

Plasma Expanders

Infusions of plasma or salt-poor albumin should be reserved for the management of life-threatening hypoalbuminemia or edema. In addition to the great expense and short supply of these blood products, their infusion only transiently reverses hypoalbuminemia in nephrotic patients because the infused protein is excreted rapidly in the urine. Albumin infusions may alleviate nephrotic edema by transiently increasing plasma oncotic pressure, thus promoting the movement of interstitial fluid into the vascular compartment. Expansion of intravascular volume also transiently reverses renal sodium retention and promotes a natriuresis.[29]

When medically indicated (e.g., in the patient with severe hypoalbuminemia and circulatory compromise), infusions of plasma expanders are optimally employed in combination with diuretic therapy. One regimen consists of infusing up to 300 ml of 15% salt-poor albumin over 45 minutes, followed by the intravenous administration of 120 mg of furosemide.[30]

Nonsteroidal Anti-inflammatory Drugs

Administration of prostaglandin-inhibiting nonsteroidal anti-inflammatory drugs may reduce urinary protein excretion in patients with nephrotic syndrome[31]; however, the so-called "antiproteinuric" response to these agents is variable. Moreover, the use of these drugs in nephrotic patients may be complicated by acute renal failure (see Chapter 3). Although most extensively described for indomethacin,[32,33] antiproteinuric effects have been reported with other nonsteroidal anti-inflammatory drugs including phenylbutazone[34] and meclofenamate.[35] Postulated mechanisms for the reduction in proteinuria mediated by these agents include: 1) alterations in intrarenal hemodynamics induced by prostaglandin inhibition, 2) direct or indirect effects on glomerular capillary permeability, and 3) interference with inflammatory mediators of glomerular injury.

There is abundant evidence that vasodilatory prostaglandins play

```
┌─────────────────────────────────────────┐
│         NEPHROTIC SYNDROME              │
│ (HEAVY PROTEINURIA, HYPOALBUMINEMIA)    │
└─────────────────────────────────────────┘
                    ⇓
       ┌──────────────────────────┐
       │ ↓ EFFECTIVE ARTERIAL VOLUME │
       └──────────────────────────┘
                    ⇓
       ┌──────────────────────────────┐
       │ ↑ ANGIOTENSIN II, ↑ CATECHOLAMINES, │
       │ ↑ ANTIDIURETIC HORMONE        │
       └──────────────────────────────┘
           ⇙                        ⇘
┌──────────────────┐  modulation   ┌────────────────────────────┐
│ ↑ KIDNEY PGE₂ and PGI₂ │ ─────────▶ │  RENAL VASOCONSTRICTION    │
└──────────────────┘              │ ↓ RENAL BLOOD FLOW, ↓ GLOMERULAR │
                                  │        FILTRATION RATE        │
                                  └────────────────────────────┘
```

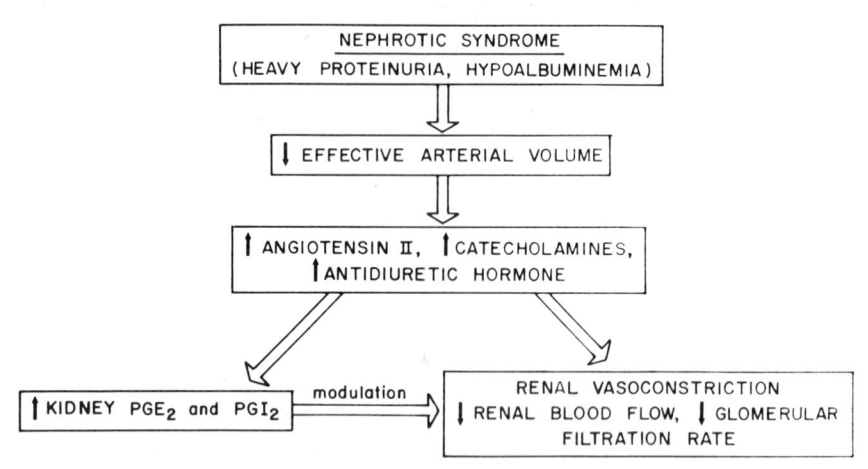

Fig 6–2.—Effects of heavy proteinuria and hypoalbuminemia on renal prostaglandin synthesis and on intrarenal hemodynamics.

important regulatory roles in the nephrotic syndrome and other conditions accompanied by a reduction in effective arterial volume.[36] Under such circumstances, PGE_2 and PGI_2 antagonize the intrarenal effect of vasoconstrictor peptides and catecholamines on the renal vasculature (Fig 6–2). Blockade of renal prostaglandin synthesis by administration of nonsteroidal anti-inflammatory drugs removes the prostaglandin-mediated vasodilatory modulation and thereby allows unopposed renal vasoconstriction. In agreement with these principles, studies of nephrotic patients demonstrate a 10% to 35% reduction in glomerular filtration rate with smaller reductions in renal blood flow after administration of indomethacin.[32, 33] These renal hemodynamic changes are accompanied by as much as 50% decrement in urinary protein excretion.[33] Although the fall in glomerular filtration rate might reduce the filtered load of protein, this is probably not the sole mechanism responsible for reduced protein excretion since the influence of indomethacin on proteinuria and on glomerular filtration rate can be dissociated in many cases. A fall in the filtration fraction might reduce proteinuria by decreasing the concentration gradient for albumin and other macromolecules at the efferent end of the glomerular capillary. It is unlikely that anti-inflammatory drugs directly alter the size or charge-selective properties of the glomerular capillary membrane; however, inhibition of prostaglandin synthesis by these agents may indirectly affect glomerular permselectivity. For example, contraction of mesangial cells by the unopposed action of angiotensin II may decrease the capillary surface available for filtration. Indomethacin and other nonsteroidal agents may block the inflammatory reaction to immunologic glomerular injury by inhibiting chemotaxis, stabilizing the lysozomes of neutrophils, or by inhibiting the production of free oxygen radicals by neutrophils and monocytes.[31] However, these effects do not account for the antiproteinuric effect of nonsteroidal anti-inflammatory drugs observed in neutrophil-independent forms of glomerular disease such as membranous glomerulopathy.

Clearly, the exact mechanisms accounting for the reduction in urinary protein excretion by nonsteroidal anti-inflammatory drugs remain to be fully defined. The antiproteinuric effect occurs early after the start of treatment and disappears rapidly after discontinuation of the drug—an observation that suggests a purely functional, hemodynamically mediated phenomenon that would be expected to have little influence on the progression of the underlying disease. Because the mechanisms leading to progressive sclerosis of glomeruli are not fully understood, it may be premature to conclude that a reduction in proteinuria does not influence the course of glomerular disease. Studies of the long-term effects of indomethacin on the course of glomerular disease have yielded conflicting results. In one retrospective review of nephrotic patients with membranoproliferative glomerulonephritis, untreated patients had a 78% ten-year mortality while patients treated with indomethacin had only a 12% ten-year mortality.[37] By contrast, a controlled study in which indomethacin was administered for two years to patients with various forms of proliferative glomerulonephritis found no appreciable difference in the rate of protein excretion after 18 months of therapy.[38]

Unfortunately, the same hemodynamic changes underlying the functional decline in proteinuria mediated by nonsteroidal anti-inflammatory drugs likely account for the potentially devastating consequences of these agents in nephrotic patients: intense renal vasoconstriction and ischemic acute renal failure. Given the hazards of nonsteroidal anti-inflammatory drugs in patients with nephrotic syndrome, these agents should be employed only when hypoalbuminemia and edema are intractably resistant to specific therapy or to more conventional supportive measures outlined above. When a drug such as indomethacin is employed in an attempt to reduce urinary protein excretion, treatment should begin with low doses and renal function should be monitored closely as the dose is gradually increased. Therapy should be discontinued if renal function declines.

Nephrectomy

The most radical approach to eliminating proteinuria is nephrectomy or destruction of remaining functioning renal tissue. The decision to perform nephrectomy in a patient with nephrotic syndrome is predicated upon the acceptability of the patient for treatment by chronic dialysis or renal transplantation. This approach should be considered only when the consequences of heavy proteinuria are incapacitating in a patient who already has significant renal failure. Nephrectomy may be performed surgically or by occluding the renal arterial supply via angiographic techniques. Nonsurgical methods for destroying renal tissue have included intramuscular injections of mercaptomerin,[39] arterial embolization with a gelatin sponge material,[40] and intrarenal injection of a rapidly hardening polymer into the renal arteries.[41]

Management of Hyperlipidemia

The controversy regarding the importance of nephrotic hyperlipidemia as a risk factor for accelerated atherosclerosis has been addressed in Chapter 3. Because hypoalbuminemia is central to the pathogenesis of nephrotic hyperlipidemia, treatment of the lipid disturbance in nephrotic syndrome is directed primarily toward elimination of proteinuria. For those patients with nephrotic syndrome resistant to specific therapy, a diet low in saturated fat may ameliorate hyperlipidemia. Clofibrate, cholestyramine, and L-tryptophan may be effective in reducing lipid levels in nephrotic patients[42]; however, the side effects and toxicities of these agents preclude their routine use in the management of nephrotic hyperlipidemia. Clofibrate toxicity is particularly prevalent among patients with nephrotic syndrome, and reflects the accumulation of high plasma levels of free clofibrate with decreased binding of the drug to albumin. A syndrome of severe proximal muscle tenderness accompanied by laboratory evidence of myonecrosis has been described in nephrotic patients receiving clofibrate.[43] It has been recommended that the daily dose of clofibrate not exceed 0.5 gm for each gram of serum albumin per deciliter.[44] Given the potential toxicity of available antilipemic drugs and the uncertainty regarding their long-term value in patients with nephrotic syndrome, these agents should probably be reserved for the treatment of severe, sustained hyperlipidemia in nephrotic patients with other risk factors for cardiovascular disease.

MANAGEMENT OF OTHER CONSEQUENCES OF HEAVY PROTEINURIA

Deficiencies of Plasma Binding Proteins

As discussed in Chapter 3, a number of hormone-binding globulins may be lost in the urine of nephrotic subjects. Plasma deficiency of thyroid-binding globulin is manifested by a high T3-resin uptake and by low levels of total T3 and T4. The free thyroxine index (i.e., the product of the T3-resin uptake and total T4) and the free levels of T3 and T4 are usually normal so that most nephrotic patients remain clinically euthyroid.[45] Measurements of free T4 and of thyroid-stimulating hormone (TSH) are the most reliable laboratory tests when hypothyroidism is suspected in patients with nephrotic syndrome.

Vitamin D deficiency and hypocalcemia resulting from urinary losses of vitamin D-binding globulin may be difficult to recognize because most hypoalbuminemic patients exhibit a reduction in total serum calcium. Measurement of a low serum ionized calcium or a low level of 1,25 dihydroxycholecalciferol are reliable clues suggesting vitamin D-binding globulin deficiency, but these tests are not available in many clinical laboratories. For practical purposes, deficiency of vitamin D-binding globulin should be suspected whenever the total serum calcium is reduced out of proportion to the reduction in serum albumin concentration.* Under such circumstances, administration of oral calcium supplements and/or vitamin D analogs should be considered.

Because transferrin has a molecular weight comparable to albumin, plasma transferrin deficiency is common in patients with nephrotic syndrome. By contrast, true iron deficiency anemia is rare because the carrying capacity of transferrin increases to keep the serum iron near normal levels.[46] Hypochromic anemia does occasionally develop when sustained transferrinuria overwhelms the compensatory increase in carrying capacity. Morever, even modest urinary losses of transferrin and iron may be sufficient to precipitate iron deficiency anemia in patients in whom iron stores are low for other reasons. Iron studies in nephrotic patients usually reveal a low serum iron level, a low total iron binding capacity, and a high saturation index. When hypochromic microcytic anemia develops in the patient

---

*As an approximation, the total serum calcium should fall no more than 0.8 mg/dl for every 1.0 gm/dl decrement in the serum albumin concentration.

with nephrotic syndrome, examination of the bone marrow for iron stores is the most reliable method for documenting iron deficiency; however, a reasonable alternative approach consists of empiric therapy with iron supplements and close follow-up to monitor the response to treatment.

The pharmacokinetics of drugs that are highly bound to albumin and other plasma proteins may be significantly altered in nephrotic patients with severe hypoalbuminemia. Because the unbound fraction is most often responsible for a drug's effect, administration of conventional doses of a highly bound drug to patients with nephrotic syndrome may result in the accumulation of unbound drug, increasing the likelihood of toxicity. At the same time, the metabolism or elimination of such drugs may be faster than usual because the drug half-life is inversely proportional to the unbound fraction. Toxicity resulting from the administration of clofibrate to nephrotic patients has been mentioned above. For any given drug, it is difficult to predict whether enhanced elimination will increase the required dose or whether reduced protein binding will decrease the dose necessary for optimal therapeutic blood levels. Whenever possible, measurement of the unbound drug concentration in plasma is the best guide to therapy.

Infection

Patients with persistent heavy proteinuria are susceptible to a variety of bacterial infections (see Chapter 3). In addition, the use of corticosteroids and other powerful immunosuppressive agents predisposes the nephrotic patient to opportunistic infections. Prophylactic antibiotics are not warranted in the routine management of patients with nephrotic syndrome; however, the physician caring for such patients should maintain a high index of suspicion and consider early antibiotic therapy with the first signs or symptoms of infection.

Encapsulated bacterial species including *Streptococcus pneumoniae* and *Hemophilus influenzae* are among the organisms most frequently encountered in patients with nephrotic syndrome.[46-48] The effectiveness of pneumococcal vaccine in preventing pneumococcal infections in this patient population has been a subject of debate. Earlier reports suggested that the vaccine may not protect against pneumococcal sepsis.[49, 50] However, a recent prospective study of children treated with polyvalent vaccine demonstrated adequate serologic conversion that conferred at least three years of protection from infection with pneumococcal types included in the vaccine, despite the concomitant administration of steroids.[51] Considering the negligible risk of this vaccine, we recommend that it be administered to all patients with persistent heavy proteinuria and the nephrotic syndrome.

Renal Vein Thrombosis

Considering the great discrepancy in the reported incidence of renal vein thrombosis among nephrotic patients, routine radiologic investigation for this potential complication of heavy proteinuria cannot be recommended for all patients with nephrotic syndrome. Until the exact risk of thromboembolism among nephrotic patients is better defined, it seems reasonable to investigate only those patients in whom clinical suspicion of renal vein thrombosis is high, i.e., those with pulmonary emboli, acute flank pain, unexplained deterioration in renal function, or new onset of hematuria.

The classical roentgenologic features of renal vein thrombosis noted with intravenous pyelography include unilateral renal enlargement, ureteral notching by collateral venous blood vessels, and pelvoclyceal irregularities. These pyelographic findings are more common in acute than in chronic renal vein thrombosis.[52] Ultrasonography[53] and computerized axial tomography[54] have been advocated for the noninvasive diagnosis of renal vein thrombosis, but selective renal venography remains the definitive diagnostic test. Small venular thrombi may be missed with venography unless concomitant venous phase arteriography is performed[27, 55]; however, the latter procedure introduces the risk of arterial puncture and enhances the risk of contrast-induced renal failure. Arteriography should be considered only when suspicion of renal vein thrombosis remains high despite a negative venogram.

Once recognized, renal vein thrombosis should be treated with anticoagulants in an attempt to preserve renal function and to prevent potentially life-threatening pulmonary emboli. It has been estimated that 40% of patients with renal vein thrombosis develop pulmonary emboli,[55] but the exact incidence of pulmonary emboli remains uncertain because many emboli are subclinical and may not be detected unless ventilation-perfusion scans are performed routinely. Results in patients with established renal vein thrombosis indicate that pulmonary embolism is virtually eliminated after anticoagulation.[53, 56, 57] Thrombectomy has been performed successfully,[58] but this potentially morbid procedure has little to offer over systemic anticoagulation.

The preferred anticoagulant drugs and the optimal duration of anticoagulant therapy for renal vein thrombosis remain subjects of debate. Heparin is often recommended for the initial management of renal vein thrombosis, but the anticoagulant efficacy of heparin in nephrotic patients has been questioned.[52] Heparin is a highly charged acidic polysaccharide that binds avidly to a number of proteins. Binding to antithrombin III rapidly activates this endogenous anticoagulant. But heparin also binds α^2-macroglobulin and may interfere with its antagonistic action on thrombin. Thus, in the presence of a low plasma concentration of antithrombin III resulting from urinary losses, heparin may theoretically promote the action of thrombin and enhance the hypercoagulable state associated with the nephrotic syndrome. Warfarin is clearly effective in the treatment of renal vein thrombosis, but its delayed onset of action usually mandates initial therapy with heparin, despite the above theoretical considerations. We prefer a regimen consisting of five to seven days of intravenous heparin overlapped and followed by a prolonged course of oral warfarin. The optimal duration of warfarin therapy has not been settled, but three to six months of treatment is probably adequate for patients in whom a sustained remission of nephrotic syndrome can be achieved. For patients with persistent nephrotic syndrome complicated by a thromboembolic event, a good case can be made for indefinite anticoagulation so long as heavy proteinuria persists. Extra care must be taken in closely monitoring the prothrombin time of nephrotic patients receiving warfarin. The drug is highly bound to serum albumin, so that frequent variations in the therapeutic dose may be required in patients with widely fluctuating serum albumin levels.

Streptokinase has been employed successfully in the management of renal vein thrombosis,[59] but there are no available studies directly comparing the benefits and risks of streptokinase and other fibrinolytic agents to conventional anticoagulant therapy. In theory, treatment with streptokinase may be less effective in patients with nephrotic syndrome than in nonproteinuric patients. The fibrinolytic action of streptokinase results from the conversion of plasminogen to plasmin, an effect that may be blunted if circulating levels of plasminogen are depleted by urinary losses of this globulin. Further clinical trials are necessary to define the role of fibrinolytic agents in the management of nephrotic patients with renal vein thrombosis.

Prospective studies are also needed to address the question of whether anticoagulants should be used prophylactically in the management of patients with persistent nephrotic syndrome. Unfortunately, there are currently no means of identifying nephrotic patients at risk for renal vein thrombosis because no single laboratory test adequately defines the hypercoagulable state that underlies their thromboembolic tendency. The beneficial effects of prophylactic warfarin therapy must be weighed against the significant risk of bleeding complications associated with prolonged anticoagulant therapy. The use of prophylactic antiplatelet agents is another approach that merits further study. As indicated in Chapter 3, platelet hyperaggregability may play an important role in the pathogenesis of thromboembolism in nephrotic syndrome. The combination of aspirin and dipyridamole has been shown to reverse the hyperaggregability of nephrotic platelets[60]; however, it remains to be proved whether antiplatelet agents can prevent thromboembolism in the nephrotic syndrome.

MANAGEMENT OF CHILDREN WITH THE NEPHROTIC SYNDROME

The consequences and complications of heavy proteinuria* in children are similar to those of adults; however, the clinical approach to the diagnosis and management of the child with nephrotic syndrome differs substantially from that in the adult patient. This difference hinges on the greater prevalence of minimal change nephropathy in children, the exquisite responsiveness of this lesion to corticosteroid therapy, and the existence of clinical criteria that accurately identify a subgroup of nephrotic children with a favorable prognosis. Given the statistical likelihood of minimal change disease in children with nephrotic syndrome, the pediatric nephrologist is less likely to perform renal biopsy and more apt to prescribe steroids empirically.

Table 6-3 shows the frequency of various histopathologic lesions underlying the nephrotic syndrome in the International Study of Kidney Disease in Children,[61] indicating a frequency of minimal change nephropathy of approximately 76% in an unselected patient population. The frequency of this lesion actually approaches 90% in children between the ages of ten months and four years.[62, 63] Among children with biopsy-proven minimal change disease, approximately 96% develop complete remission from proteinuria with steroid therapy, most often within three to four weeks. Following an initial complete remis-

---

*In children, nephrotic range proteinuria is defined as >40 mg of protein per square meter of body surface area per hour or >50 mg of protein per kilogram of body weight per day.

sion, as many as 85% of children have subsequent relapses[63] requiring additional courses of corticosteroids or treatment with alkylating agents such as cyclophosphamide or chlorambucil.[64, 65]

A number of clinical criteria define a subgroup of children with a favorable response to steroid therapy and allow the surprisingly accurate prediction of underlying minimal change nephropathy. The criteria for inclusion in this favorable subgroup are listed in Table 6–4 and include 1) ages 10 months to 8 years, 2) absence of azotemia, 3) absence of hematuria, 4) absence of hypertension, 5) normal serum concentration of C3, and 6) highly selective proteinuria. Approximately 95% of such patients have minimal change disease, response to steroid therapy, and have a favorable prognosis.[66] Low serum levels of the third component of complement (C3) usually indicate the presence of membranoproliferative glomerulonephritis; however, low levels can be associated with the nephrotic syndrome in systemic lupus erythematosus, post-infectious glomerulonephritis, and various vasculitides. As indicated in Table 6–4, a clear response to steroids is not seen in nephrotic children with C3 levels less than 100 mg/dl. The selectivity index can be quite helpful diagnostically in children. Among patients with biopsy-proven minimal change disease, highly selective proteinuria (defined as an IgG/transferring clearance ratio of less than 0.10) has been detected in approximately 70% of cases.[62, 63] Conversely, 96% of nephrotic children with a selectivity index less than 0.1 have minimal change disease on biopsy.[66] Thus, the finding of highly selective proteinuria is a sensitive predictor of minimal change disease in children, but the detection of poorly selective proteinuria does not exclude this diagnosis.

TABLE 6–3.—DISTRIBUTION OF CHILDREN WITH NEPHROTIC SYNDROME BY HISTOPATHOLOGY*

CATEGORY	NO. OF PATIENTS	%
Minimal change nephrotic syndrome	398	76.4
Membranoproliferative glomerulonephritis	39	7.5
Focal and segmental glomerulosclerosis	36	6.5
Proliferative glomerulonephritis	12	2.3
Pure diffuse mesangial proliferation	12	2.3
Focal and global glomerulosclerosis	9	1.5
Membranous glomerulophropathy	8	1.5
Chronic glomerulonephritis	3	0.6
Unclassified	4	0.8
Total	**521**	**100.0**

*Reprinted from *Kidney International* (Vol. 13:159–165, 1978) with permission.

TABLE 6-4.—CLINICAL PREDICTION OF
RESPONSE TO STEROID THERAPY IN CHILDREN
WITH NEPHROTIC SYNDROME*

CRITERIA	COMPLETE RESPONSE (%)
Pathology	
Minimal change lesion	96
Other	7
Selective protein index	
<0.1	97
<0.2	92
>0.2	32
Complement (C3)	
<100 mg/dl	0
>100 mg/dl	75
Hematuria	
Present	33
Absent	87
Age	
<10 mo.	10
10 mo–3 yr	91
3–8 yr	75
8–17 yr	45
Hypertension	
Present	33
Absent	78
Azotemia	
Present	36
Absent	78

*Courtesy of Grupe W.E.: *Postgraduate Medicine* 65:229, 1979.

Given the above considerations, renal biopsy is generally reserved for the evaluation of nephrotic children in whom the clinical criteria outlined above suggest a histopathologic entity other than minimal change disease. In addition, biopsy may be warranted in the rare child who fails to respond to steroid therapy despite favorable clinical indices. Studies of children with glomerular lesions traditionally regarded as "steroid-unresponsive" (e.g., focal glomerulosclerosis) suggest that a subset of such patients actually respond favorably to corticosteroids.[67] Thus, a good case can be made for an initial empirical trial of steroids in all children with idiopathic nephrotic syndrome, regardless of associated clinical findings. Using this approach, renal biopsy would be considered only for those children who fail to respond to steroids.

REFERENCES

1. King S.E.: Albuminuria (proteinuria) in renal diseases: II. Preliminary observations on the clinical course of patients with orthostatic albuminuria. *N.Y. State J. Med.* 59:825, 1959.

2. Thompson A.L., Durrett R.R., Robinson R.R.: Fixed and reproducible orthostatic proteinuria: VI. Results of a 10-year follow-up evaluation. *Ann. Intern. Med.* 73:236, 1970.
3. Springberg P.D., Garrett L.E., Thompson A.L., et al.: Fixed and reproducible orthostatic proteinuria: Results of a 20-year follow-up study. *Ann. Intern. Med.* 97:516, 1982.
4. Abuelo J.G.: Proteinuria: diagnostic principles and procedures. *Ann. Intern. Med.* 98:186, 1983.
5. Robinson R.R., Glover S.N., Phillipi P.J., et al.: Fixed and reproducible orthostatic proteinuria: I. Light microscopic studies of the kidney. *Am. J. Pathol.* 39:291, 1961.
6. Phillip P.J., Reynolds, J., Yamauchi H., et al.: Persistent proteinuria in asymptomatic individuals: Renal biopsy study on 50 patients. *Milit. Med.* 131:1311, 1966.
7. Torres V.E., Velosa J.A., Holley K.E., et al.: The progression of vesicoureteral reflux nephropathy. *Ann. Intern. Med.* 92:776, 1980.
8. Mogensen C.E.: Long-term antihypertensive treatment inhibiting progression of diabetic nephropathy. *Br. Med. J.* 285:685, 1982.
9. Parving H., Anderson A.R., Smidt U.M., et al.: Early aggressive antihypertensive treatment reduces rate of decline in kidney function in diabetic nephropathy. *Lancet* 1:2275, 1983.
10. Takekoshi Y., Shida N., Saheki Y., et al.: Strong association between membranous nephropathy and hepatitis-B surface antigenaemia in Japanese children. *Lancet* 2:1065, 1978.
11. Rao T.K., Nicastri A.O., Frideman E.A.: Natural history of heroin-associated nephropathy. *N. Engl. J. Med.* 290:19, 1974.
12. Treser G., Cherubin C., Lonergan E.T., et al.: Renal lesions in narcotic addicts. *Am. J. Med.* 57:687, 1974.
13. Pardo V., Strauss J., Kramer H., et al.: Nephropathy associated with sickle cell anemia: An autologous immune complex nephritis. II. Clinicopathologic study of seven patients. *Am. J. Med.* 59:650, 1975.
14. World M.J.: Variables discriminating between cryptogenic glomerular lesions in adults with the nephrotic syndrome. *Q. J. Med.* 45:451, 1976.
15. Shearn M.A.: Normocholesterolemic nephrotic syndrome of systemic lupus erythematosus. *Am. J. Med. Sci.* 242:211, 1962.
16. Cameron J.S.: Histology, protein clearances and response to treatment in the nephrotic syndrome. *Br. Med. J.* 4:352, 1968.
17. Lee J.C., Yamauchi H., Hopper J.: The association of cancer and the nephrotic syndrome. *Ann. Intern. Med.* 64:41, 1966.
18. Row P.G., Cameron J.S., Turner D.R., et al.: Membranous nephropathy: Long-term follow-up and association with neoplasia. *Q. J. Med.* 44:207, 1975.
19. Kaplan B.S., Klassen J., Gault M.H.: Glomerular injury in patients with neoplasia. *Annu. Rev. Med.* 27:117, 1976.
20. Eagen J., Lewis E.J.: Glomerulopathies of neoplasia. *Kidney Int.* 11:297, 1977.
21. Iverson P., Brun C.: Aspiration biopsy of the kidney. *Am. J. Med.* 11:324, 1951.
22. Kark R.M., Muehrcke R.C.: Biopsy of the kidney in the prone position. *Lancet* 1:1047, 1954.
23. Gault M.H., Muehrcke R.C.: Renal biopsy: Current views and controversies. *Nephron* 34:1, 1983.
24. Klatky M.A.: Is renal biopsy necessary in adults with nephrotic syndrome? *Lancet* 2:1264, 1983.
25. Kassirer J.P.: Is renal biopsy necessary for optimal management of the idiopathic nephrotic syndrome: *Kidney Int.* 24:561, 1983.
26. Blainey J.D.: High protein diets in the treatment of the nephrotic syndrome. *Clin. Sci.* 13:567, 1954.
27. Wagoner R.D.: *The Nephrotic Syndrome: Discussions in Patient Management.* New York, Medical Examination Publishing Co., 1981.

28. Earley L.E.: Edema formation and the use of diuretics. *Calif. Med.* 114:56, 1971.
29. Grausz H., Lieberman R., Earley L.E.: Effect of plasma albumin on sodium reabsorption in patients with nephrotic syndrome. *Kidney Int.* 1:47, 1972.
30. Davison A.M., Lambie A.T.: Salt-poor albumin in the management of nephrotic syndrome. *Br. Med. J.* 1:481, 1974.
31. Michielsen P., Varenterghem Y.: Proteinuria and nonsteroidal anti-inflammatory drugs. *Adv. Nephrol.* 12:139, 1983.
32. Arisz L., Donker A.J.M., Brentjens J.R., et al.: The effect of indomethacin on proteinuria and kidney function in the nephrotic syndrome. *Acta Med. Scand.* 199:121, 1976.
33. Tiggeler R., Hulme B., Wijdeveld P.: Effect of indomethacin on glomerular permeability in the nephrotic syndrome. *Kidney Int.* 16:312, 1979.
34. Feischi A., Bianchi V., Ghirado G.: Results of treatment with phenylbutazone in albuminuric syndromes, in Garattni S., Dukes M.N.G. (eds.): *Nonsteroidal Antiinflammatory Drugs*. Amsterdam, Excerpta Medica International Congress Series, 1965, vol. 82, p. 437.
35. Torres V.E., Velosa J.A., Holley K.E., et al.: Mezlofenemate treatment of recurrent idiopathic nephrotic syndrome with focal glomerulosclerosis after renal transplantation. *Mayo Clin. Proc.* 59:146, 1984.
36. Dunn M.J.: Nonsteroidal anti-inflammatory drugs and renal function. *Annu. Rev. Med.* 35:411, 1984.
37. Michielsen P., Varenterghen Y., Roels L.: Treatment of chronic glomerulonephritis with indomethacin, in Kluthe R., Vogt A., Batsford S.R. (eds.): *Glomerulonephritis*. New York, John Wiley, & Sons, 1977.
38. Rose G.: Medical Research Council Trials, in Kluthe R., Vogt A., Batsford S.R. (eds.): *Glomerulonephritis*. New York, John Wiley & Sons, 1977.
39. Avram M.M., Lipner H.I., Gan A.C.: Medical nephrectomy. The use of metallic salts for the control of massive proteinuria in the nephrotic syndrome. *Trans. Am. Soc. Artif. Intern. Organs* 22:431, 1976.
40. McCarron D.A., Rubin R.J., Barnes B.A.: Therapeutic bilateral renal infarction in end-stage renal disease. *N. Engl. J. Med.* 294:652, 1976.
41. Henrich W.L., Goldman M., Dotter C.T., et al.: Therapeutic renal arterial occlusion for elimination of proteinuria—medical nephrectomy. *Arch. Intern. Med.* 136:840, 1976.
42. Schapel G.J., Edwards K.D., Nearle F.C.: Factorial study of the efficacy of cholestyrameine, L-tryptophan and clofibrate in human nephrotic hyperlipidaemia. *Prog. Biochem. Pharmacol.* 9:82, 1974.
43. Bridgman J.F., Rosen S.M., Thorp J.M.: Complications during clofibrate treatment of nephrotic syndrome hyperlipoproteinuria. *Lancet* 2:506, 1972.
44. Earley L.E.: The nephrotic syndrome, in Earley L.E., Gottshalk C.W. (eds.): *Strauss and Welt's Diseases of the Kidney*. Boston, Little, Brown & Co., 1979, p. 800.
45. Afrasiabi M.A., Vaxiri N.D., Grinue G., et al.: Thyroid function studies in the nephrotic syndrome. *Ann. Intern. Med.* 90:355, 1979.
46. Arneil G.C.: 164 children with nephritis. *Lancet* 22:1103, 1961.
47. Rubin H.M., Blair E.B., Michaels R.H.: Hemophilus and pneumococcal peritonitis in children with nephrotic syndrome. *Pediatrics* 56:598, 1975.
48. Rusthover J., Kabins S.A.: Hemophilus influenzae F cellulitis with bacteremia, peritonitis and pleuritis in an adult with nephrotic syndrome. *South. Med. J.* 71:1443, 1978.
49. Primack W.A., Rosel M., Thirumoorthi M.C., et al.: Failure of pneumococcal vaccine to prevent Streptococcus pneumoniae sepsis in nephrotic children. *Lancet* 2:1192, 1979.
50. Moore D.H., Shackelford P.C., Robson A.M., et al.: Recurrent pneumococcal sepsis and defective opsonization after pneumococcal capsular polysaccharide vaccine in a child with nephrotic syndrome. *J. Pediatr.* 46:882, 1980.

51. Wilkes J.C., Nelson J.D., Worthen H.G., et al.: Response to pneumococcal vaccination in children with nephrotic syndrome. *Am. J. Kidney Dis.* 2:43, 1982.
52. Llach F., Papper S., Massry S.G.: The clinical spectrum of renal vein thrombosis: Acute and chronic. *Am. J. Med.* 69:819, 1980.
53. Rosenfield A.T., Zeman R.K., Cronan J., et al.: Ultrasound in experimental and clinical renal vein thrombosis. *Radiology* 137:735, 1980.
54. Zerhouni E.A., Barth K.H., Siegelman S.S.: Demonstration of venous thrombosis by computed tomography. *A.J.R.* 134:753, 1980.
55. Llach F.: Nephrotic syndrome: hypercoagulability, renal vein thrombosis and other thromboembolic complications, in Brenner B.M., Stein J.H. (eds.): *Contemporary Issues in Nephrology: Nephrotic Syndrome.* New York, Churchill Livingstone, Inc., 1982, vol. 9, pp. 121–144.
56. Harrington J.T., Kassirer J.P.: Renal venous thrombosis. *Annu. Rev. Med.* 33:255, 1982.
57. Rosemann E., Pollack V.E., Pirani C.C.: Renal vein thrombosis in the adult. A clinical and pathologic study based on renal biopsies. *Medicine* 47:269, 1968.
58. Fein R.L., Chart A., Leviton A.: Renal vein thrombectomy for treatment of renal vein thrombosis associated with the nephrotic syndrome. *J. Urol.* 99:1, 1968.
59. Crowley J.P., Matarese R.A., Quevedo S.F., et al.: Fibrinolytic therapy for bilateral renal vein thrombosis. *Arch. Intern. Med.* 144:159, 1984.
60. Andrassy K., Ritz E., Bonner J.: Hypercoagulability in the nephrotic syndrome. *Klin. Wochenschr.* 58:1029, 1980.
61. International Study of Kidney Disease in Children: Nephrotic syndrome in children: prediction of histopathology from clinical and laboratory characteristics at time of diagnosis. *Kidney Int.* 13:159, 1978.
62. White R.H.R., Glasgow E.F., Mills R.J.: Clinicopathological study of nephrotic syndrome in childhood. *Lancet* 1:1353, 1970.
63. Makker S.P., Heymann W.: The idiopathic nephrotic syndrome of childhood: A clinical reevaluation of 148 cases. *Am. J. Dis. Child.* 127:830, 1974.
64. McCory W.W., Shibuya M., Lu W.H., et al.: Therapeutic and toxic effects observed with different dosage programs of cyclophosphamide in treatment of steroid-responsive but frequently relapsing nephrotic syndrome. *J. Pediatr.* 82:614, 1973.
65. Grupe W.E., Makker S.P., Ingelfinger J.R.: Chlorambucil treatment of frequently relapsing nephrotic syndrome in childhood. *Pediatr. Res.* 11:560, 1977.
66. Grupe W.E.: Relapsing nephrotic syndrome in childhood. *Kidney Int.* 16:75, 1979.
67. Arbus G.S., Poucell S., Bacheyie G.S., et al.: Focal segmental glomerulosclerosis with idiopathic nephrotic syndrome: three types of clinical response. *J. Pediatr.* 101:40, 1982.

7 *Illustrative Cases*

IN THIS CHAPTER we present case histories to illustrate principles in the diagnosis and management of patients with proteinuria. Pertinent information from the history and physical examination and selected laboratory measurements are given. A series of comments accompanies each case. When appropriate, the reader will be referred to earlier chapters for explanation of the clinical points illustrated.

PATIENT 1. A WOMAN WITH CONGESTIVE HEART FAILURE AND NEPHROTIC SYNDROME

A 59-year-old woman was admitted to the hospital because of weight gain, peripheral edema, and dyspnea. One year earlier she was hospitalized for an acute myocardial infarction complicated by congestive heart failure. She subsequently received digitalis and furosemide. Six months prior to admission, physical examination was remarkable only for 1+ pedal edema. Laboratory studies at that time revealed a BUN of 32 mg/dl, and serum creatinine concentration of 1.7 mg/dl. Dipstick of a urine specimen revealed 1+ protein. A 24-hour urine specimen contained 340 mg of protein.

Six weeks prior to admission, the patient complained of intermittent right knee pain. An x-ray of the knee showed changes compatible with osteoarthritis. Fenoprofen was prescribed and the knee pain improved. Subsequently, the patient noted a 15-lb weight gain associated with edema of the ankles and hands. For three days prior to admission she noted progressively increasing dyspnea on exertion.

On physical examination she appeared to be in modest respiratory distress. Blood pressure was 140/90 mm Hg, and respirations were 24/minute. An S_3 gallop was present. There were decreased breath sounds and dullness to percussion at the right lung base. There was 3+ pitting edema of both legs to the mid-thighs and periorbital edema was present.

Comments: This patient's presenting symptoms were compatible with worsening congestive heart failure. However, admission laboratory data revealed that she had acute renal insufficiency and heavy proteinuria accompanied by hypoalbuminemia. Administration of

ADMISSION LABORATORY DATA, PATIENT 1	
BUN	89 mg/dl
Creatinine	7.2 mg/dl
Sodium	130 mEq/L
Potassium	5.1 mEq/L
Chloride	91 mEq/L
Bicarbonate	20 mEq/L
Albumin	1.9 gm/dl
Chest x-ray	Cardiomegaly; large right pleural effusion
ECG	Old anterior infarction; no new ischemic changes
Urinalysis	Dipstick: 4+ protein Microscopic examination: 10–15 white blood cells per high power field; occasional white blood cell casts; rare renal tubular cells.

prostaglandin-inhibiting nonsteroidal anti-inflammatory drugs such as fenoprofen to patients with congestive heart failure may cause a functional reduction in glomerular filtration rate, but this phenomenon alone does not account for the patient's proteinuria and hypoalbuminemia. Furthermore, the presence of white blood cell casts in the urine sediment strongly suggests renal parenchymal injury. As discussed in Chapter 1, functional proteinuria commonly accompanies congestive heart failure, but rarely accounts for more than 1 to 2 gm of urinary protein per day. This patient probably had functional proteinuria six months prior to admission; however, the 4+ dipstick reading and hypoalbuminemia at the time of admission strongly suggest that she had developed a glomerular disease.

Six hundred milliliters of a transudative right pleural effusion were removed by thoracentesis and the patient's dyspnea rapidly improved. Dietary sodium restriction was instituted and the patient received daily intravenous furosemide. During the first five hospital days, a 10-lb weight loss ensued, but the patient's serum creatinine concentration gradually rose to 9.5 mg/dl. The serum sodium concentration on the fifth hospital day was 128 mEq/L. A 24-hour urine specimen obtained on the second hospital day revealed 11.3 gm of protein. The serum cholesterol was 220 mg/dl and the serum triglyceride 195 mg/dl.

Comments: The development of nephrotic syndrome in this patient with a history of cardiac failure led to renal sodium retention with further decompensation of left ventricular function. Congestive heart failure, the nephrotic syndrome, and acute renal insufficiency likely account for her hyponatremia; however, in this setting, measurement of serum lipid levels was helpful in excluding "pseudohyponatremia" due to nephrotic hyperlipidemia. As discussed in Chapter 6, hyponatremia in the patient with nephrotic syndrome may reflect intravascular volume depletion. Under such circumstances, diuretics must be

Illustrative Cases

administered with great caution to avoid further contraction of extracellular volume. In this case, a successful diuresis may have occurred at the expense of a further decline in renal function.

On the sixth hospital day, a percutaneous renal biopsy was performed. By light microscopy, the glomeruli appeared normal. The renal interstitium was densely infiltrated with lymphocytes and plasma cells. Electron microscopic examination of glomerular capillary membranes revealed foot process fusion. On the basis of the biopsy results, fenoprofen nephrotoxicity was suspected, and the drug was discontinued. The patient required three hemodialyses during the subsequent week but then exhibited a gradual resolution of azotemia and heavy proteinuria. One month after discharge from the hospital, the serum creatinine concentration was 1.9 mg/dl and a 24-hour specimen contained 400 mg of protein.

Comments: This case is an example of a unique syndrome of acute renal failure and nephrotic proteinuria that has been associated with the use of fenoprofen and other nonsteroidal anti-inflammatory drugs. The pathophysiology of this syndrome has not been fully elucidated; however, surface marker analyses of cells within the interstitial infiltrate indicate a preponderance of cytotoxic T-cells, suggesting a cell-mediated hypersensitivity reaction (see Chapter 4). Because pathologic changes in the glomeruli are limited to foot process fusion, pathologists have referred to this entity as "interstitial nephritis with minimal change disease." It has been suggested that foot process fusion and heavy proteinuria may be mediated by a lymphokine produced by sensitized lymphocytes. Once recognized, the treatment of choice consists of discontinuing the offending agent.

PATIENT 2. A MAN WITH FLANK PAIN AND GROSS HEMATURIA

A 65-year-old man was hospitalized for evaluation of sudden left flank pain associated with gross hematuria. Two weeks earlier he had complained of ankle swelling. Physical examination at that time revealed 1+ pedal edema. Bumetanide was prescribed empirically and the patient's edema resolved within two days. Three days prior to admission, the patient developed lightheadedness upon standing. On the evening of admission he noted the sudden onset of a sharp pain in the left flank and came to the emergency room where he passed grossly bloody urine.

On physical examination, blood pressure was 110/70 mm Hg in the supine position and 90/50 mm Hg in the standing position. Skin turgor was poor with marked tenting of the skin over the anterior thighs. There was exquisite tenderness to percussion over the left costovertebral angle. Peripheral edema was not detected. The presumptive diagnoses in the emergency room were (1) diuretic-induced volume depletion, and (2) ureterolithiasis.

ADMISSION LABORATORY DATA, PATIENT 2	
BUN	46 mg/dl
Creatinine	1.3 mg/dl
Hematocrit	56%
Platelet Count	364,000
PT, PTT	Normal
KUB	No calcifications seen
Urinalysis	Specific gravity 1.028; Dipstick 4+ blood, 4+ protein
	Microscopic examination: red blood cells too numerous to count; no cellular casts.

The patient received intravenous normal saline and his orthostatic hypotension resolved. Bumetanide was discontinued. Intravenous pyelography was performed the following morning and revealed no evidence of ureterolithiasis. The right kidney measured 11 cm in length and the left kidney 16 cm. Marked notching of the left ureter suggested renal venous collaterals and a radiologic diagnosis of left renal vein thrombosis was entertained. A renal venogram was performed the following day and confirmed the presence of a large clot in the left renal vein with extension into the inferior vena cava.

Comments: Although ureterolithiasis was a tenable diagnosis in this patient with flank pain and hematuria, the radiologic studies suggested renal vein thrombosis complicating heavy proteinuria. Interpretation of this patient's dipstick test for proteinuria was clouded by the knowledge that patients with gross hematuria may exhibit false-positive tests for proteinuria (see Chapter 1). In this setting, the diagnosis of nephrotic syndrome should be corroborated by quantitation of 24-hour urinary protein excretion and by measurement of the serum albumin concentration.

As discussed in Chapter 3, renal vein thrombosis in patients with nephrotic syndrome reflects a generalized tendency to develop thromboembolism resulting from a hypercoagulable state. The injudicious use of potent diuretics may enhance this hypercoagulable state by inducing extracellular volume contraction and hemoconcentration. Had nephrotic syndrome been recognized as the cause of this patient's mild pedal edema two weeks prior to admission, a trial of dietary sodium restriction would have been preferable to the administration of a potent loop diuretic.

A 24-hour urine specimen contained 5.6 gm of protein. The serum albumin was 2.9 gm/dl at the time of admission but fell to 2.2 gm/dl following rehydration. A ventilation-perfusion scan of the lungs was normal. Intravenous heparin was administered for seven days and the patient's flank pain and hematuria resolved. Oral warfarin was subsequently prescribed and the patient was discharged on the 11th hospital day. The discharge diagnosis was idiopathic nephrotic syndrome complicated by renal vein thrombosis. Because percutaneous biopsy could not be performed while the patient was receiving anticoagulants, prednisone 120 mg q.o.d. was administered empirically for two months. Six weeks following discharge from the hospital, 24-hour urinary protein excretion had fallen to 110 mg and the serum albumin concentration was normal. Warfarin therapy was discontinued after a six-month course. Two months later the patient again developed heavy proteinuria and edema. Renal biopsy at that time revealed minimal change nephropathy.

Comments: As discussed in Chapter 6, the role of renal biopsy in the management of patients with idiopathic nephrotic syndrome has been the subject of increasing controversy. Considering the relatively low risk of alternate day steroid therapy, we believe that an empiric trial of prednisone is reasonable when relative or absolute contraindications preclude renal biopsy. In this case, the major rationale for "blind" steroid therapy was the concern that the patient would continue to exhibit a thromboembolic tendency with persistent heavy proteinuria.

A wide variety of glomerular lesions, including minimal change nephropathy, has been associated with thromboembolic disease. In adult patients with nephrotic syndrome, membranous glomerulopathy is the histologic lesion most frequently associated with renal vein thrombosis. None of the clinical features of this case, including the patient's presentation with renal vein thrombosis and his response to steroid therapy, was sufficiently discriminating to allow an accurate prediction of the underlying glomerular histopathology.

PATIENT 3. A CHILD WITH FREQUENTLY RELAPSING NEPHROTIC SYNDROME

A 9-year-old boy was referred to a pediatric nephrologist for management of nephrotic syndrome. The child's mother noted a three-week history of in-

LABORATORY DATA, PATIENT 3	
BUN	9 mg/dl
Creatinine	0.6 mg/dl
CH50, C3, C4	Normal
ANA	Negative
Urinalysis	Dipstick: 3+ protein, 0 blood
	Microscopic examination: free lipid droplets and occasional oval fat bodies
24-hour urine protein	3.1 gm
Selectivity Index	0.18

creasing abdominal girth and periorbital puffiness that was most notable upon waking in the morning. On physical examination, the boy weighed 27 kg. Blood pressure was 88/60 mm Hg. Abdominal examination revealed shifting dullness consistent with ascites. There was marked periorbital edema and 1+ ankle edema.

Comments: Minimal change nephropathy accounts for more than 70% of cases of idiopathic nephrotic syndrome in children and thus represents the statistically likely diagnosis in this boy. The patient's age, the absence of hypertension and azotemia, and the normal serum complement levels are clinical features that predict a favorable response to steroid therapy (see Chapter 6). However, the selectivity index was within an intermediate range. Under these circumstances, most pediatric nephrologists would avoid renal biopsy and treat the patient empirically with steroids for a presumptive diagnosis of minimal change disease.

The patient received prednisone 1 mg/kg on a daily basis. Three weeks after initiating this therapy a complete remission ensued. After two months of treatment, prednisone was gradually tapered and discontinued. During the subsequent 13 months, nephrotic syndrome recurred on four occasions. With each of the first three relapses, complete remission was achieved with prednisone. A 12-week trial of chlorambucil and prednisone was begun following the fourth relapse. While receiving this combination of medications, the patient's blood pressure gradually increased to 130/90 mm Hg. The serum creatinine concentration, previously within a normal range, increased to 1.6 mg/dl. A percutaneous renal biopsy revealed focal and segmental glomerulosclerosis.

Comments: The development of hypertension and azotemia is distinctly unusual among patients with minimal change nephropathy. A small percentage of patients with the typical clinical features or morphological findings of minimal change disease may display steroid resistance, and some pursue an atypical course with progressive renal insufficiency. In such cases, renal biopsy usually reveals previously unrecognized structural glomerular disease, most commonly focal glomerulosclerosis. It remains unclear whether minimal change disease and focal glomerulosclerosis are distinct clinicopathologic entities or whether progression to focal glomerulosclerosis may be one pathway taken by a small number of patients with minimal change disease and frequently relapsing nephrotic syndrome.

The appearance of hypertension frequently heralds the onset of renal insufficiency in patients with focal glomerulosclerosis. Because approximately 50% of patients with focal glomerulosclerosis develop end-state renal failure within ten years of diagnosis, this child's prognosis remains guarded.

PATIENT 4. A COLLEGE STUDENT WITH INTERMITTENT PROTEINURIA

As part of a college entrance physical examination, an 18-year-old man had a urinalysis that revealed 2+ protein. Three years earlier, the patient's pediatrician asked him to have a repeat urinalysis after discovering a "trace of protein" in his urine, but the subsequent urinalysis was reportedly normal. The patient appeared to be in excellent health and denied the use of any medications. His physical examination was entirely unremarkable.

Comments: This patient's history suggests intermittent proteinuria. Based on the history and physical examination, there was no obvious cause of functional proteinuria and no apparent systemic disease associated with enhanced urinary protein excretion. This patient should be tested for true postural proteinuria (see Chapter 6), because its discovery implies a favorable prognosis and influences the extent and frequency of follow-up examinations.

The patient was instructed in the collection of recumbent and upright urine collections during a 24-hour period. A nine-hour recumbent urine specimen contained 30 mg of protein. A 15-hour upright urine contained 400 mg of protein. The patient was instructed to have annual physical examinations in the college's health service and to submit recumbent and upright urine specimens for each examination. Four years later, the patient's recumbent urinary protein excretion remained within normal limits, and protein excretion in a 14-hour upright collection had declined to 100 mg.

Comments: This young man's clinical course is typical of patients with true postural proteinuria. Most long-term studies of patients with this pattern of proteinuria suggest that excessive urinary protein excretion gradually remits with time (see Chapters 1 and 6). Although some patients with postural proteinuria have minor histologic glomerular abnormalities, renal biopsy is not warranted in the routine management of such patients because no specific therapy is warranted. The prognosis of this patient is excellent and the likelihood of his developing renal insufficiency is extremely small.

LABORATORY DATA, PATIENT 4	
BUN	15 mg/dl
Creatinine	0.9 mg/dl
Creatinine clearance	128/ml/min
Urinalysis	Dipstick: 2+ protein, 0 blood, 0 glucose
	Specific gravity: 1.009
	Microscopic examination: Normal
24-hour urine protein	750 mg

PATIENT 5. A WOMAN WITH RHEUMATOID ARTHRITIS AND HEAVY PROTEINURIA

A 49-year-old woman with longstanding rheumatoid arthritis was hospitalized for percutaneous renal biopsy. She first developed symmetrical polyarthritis involving the hands, wrists, and knees at age 36. At that time, rheumatoid factor was positive at a titer of 1:2560, and a test for antinuclear antibodies was negative. She initially responded well to salicylate therapy. During the subsequent ten years, she had numerous exacerbations and remissions of arthritis. In addition to several courses of salicylate therapy, she admitted to using a variety of "over-the-counter" combination analgesics.

By the age of 46, she had developed several subcutaneous rheumatoid nodules and exhibited notable deformities of the wrists and knees. She received an eight-month trial of gold therapy with little objective improvement. While receiving gold injections, her renal function and urinary protein excretion were monitored closely and remained normal. Gold therapy was abandoned when the patient developed a severe flare of arthritis at age 47, requiring hospitalization and a brief course of steroids.

She subsequently received penicillamine with significant symptomatic improvement and objective abatement of her arthritis. After five months of penicillamine therapy, 2+ proteinuria was first detected in a monthly urinalysis. At that time, a 24-hour urine specimen contained 1200 mg of protein. The dose of penicillamine was reduced by approximately 25%, and a repeat 24-hour urine specimen one month later revealed 800 mg of protein. During the subsequent year, serial monthly urine specimens revealed a gradual increase in urinary protein excretion to 2.5 gm per day. Penicillamine was discontinued. Four months later, urinary protein excretion had increased to 4.1 gm per day.

On physical examination blood pressure was 130/80 mm Hg. There were multiple subcutaneous nodules on the extensor surfaces of both arms. There was synovial thickening of the wrist, knee, and proximal interphalangeal joints. There was no detectable peripheral edema.

Comments: Although this patient had heavy proteinuria, she did not exhibit other features of the nephrotic syndrome, i.e., hypoalbuminemia, edema, hyperlipidemia, or lipiduria. Nevertheless, urinary

ADMISSION LABORATORY DATA, PATIENT 5	
BUN	22 mg/dl
Creatinine	1.6 mg/dl
Electrolytes	Normal
Albumin	3.9 gm/dl
Cholesterol, Triglycerides	Normal
ANA	Negative
Cryoglobulins	None detected
24-hour urine protein	4.3 gm
Urinalysis	Dipstick: 3+ protein, 0 blood, 0 glucose Microscopic examination: rare granular casts, no lipids noted.

excretion of more than 3 gm of protein virtually assured the presence of an underlying glomerulopathy (see Chapter 1).

A number of glomerular diseases merit consideration in this case. Although rheumatoid arthritis is a disease mediated, in part, by circulating immune-complexes, it is of interest that immune-complex mediated glomerulonephritis is not a regular feature of rheumatoid arthritis in the absence of rheumatoid vasculitis. Whenever a patient with rheumatoid arthritis develops evidence of renal disease, systemic lupus erythematosus should be excluded, since the two diseases may coexist. Mixed cryoglobulinemia is an occasional cause of glomerulonephritis in patients with rheumatoid arthritis, but occurs more commonly in patients who also have Sjögren's syndrome.

Treatment regimens for patients with rheumatoid arthritis include a number of drugs that can cause glomerular disease. The chronic use of combination analgesics, especially those containing aspirin and phenacetin, has been associated with interstitial nephritis, papillary necrosis, and progressive renal insufficiency. In its advanced stages, this predominantly interstitial disease may be accompanied by secondary focal glomerulosclerosis and heavy proteinuria. Nephrotic syndrome complicating analgesic abuse usually occurs in patients with advanced azotemia, making analgesic nephropathy an unlikely diagnosis in this case.

Treatment with gold and/or penicillamine has been associated with proteinuria and the nephrotic syndrome (see Chapter 4). The glomerular lesion induced by these drugs most commonly resembles idiopathic membranous glomerulopathy. Although most rheumatologists suggest that gold salts be discontinued in patients who develop proteinuria, opinions vary regarding the need to discontinue penicillamine when proteinuria complicates its use. Given the disabling nature of the disease being treated, many physicians elect to continue to drug, sometimes at reduced doses, as long as proteinuria remains mild and asymptomatic.

Light microscopic examination of the renal biopsy specimen revealed large nodules in all glomeruli. Using a Congo red stain, these nodules exhibited green birefringence when viewed under polarized light. Electron microscopic examination of the glomerular nodules revealed fibrillar structures compatible with amyloidosis.

Comments: Rheumatoid arthritis, chronic osteomyelitis, and tuberculosis are the most common inflammatory/infectious diseases associated with secondary amyloidosis (see Chapter 4). Heavy proteinuria and other manifestations of secondary amyloidosis sometimes remit with treatment of the underlying disease. Given the progressive nature of this patient's rheumatoid arthritis, her renal prognosis is grim and the likelihood of continued proteinuria and progressive renal insufficiency is great.

PATIENT 6. A YOUNG MAN WITH HODGKIN'S DISEASE AND NEPHROTIC SYNDROME

A 23-year-old man was hospitalized for evaluation of fever, night sweats, and anasarca. For eight months prior to admission, he noted anorexia associated with a 30-lb weight loss. Three months prior to admission he first developed edema of the ankles that progressed to involve his abdominal wall and arms. He subsequently noted nightly fevers and drenching night sweats. He initially refused to seek medical care but ultimately was brought to the Emergency Room by his wife when he became acutely confused and lethargic.

On physical examination, blood pressure was 70/50 mm Hg, temperature 38.3 C°, pulse 120/minute, respirations 20/minute. The patient was alert but disoriented. There was a 4×5-cm firm and immobile mass in the left supraclavicular area. The spleen was palapable 4 cm below the left costal margin. There was 3+ pitting edema present in the legs, arms, abdomen and chest.

Comments: This patient with nephrotic syndrome presented with hypotension and prerenal azotemia, suggesting a profound reduction in effective arterial volume. Under these circumstances, infusion of albumin and concomitant administration of diuretics is warranted to prevent further circulatory compromise. The elevated sedimentation rate in this case is difficult to interpret. Although compatible with a lymphoproliferative malignancy or systemic infection, a high sedimentation rate is also commonly observed in nephrotic patients, presumably resulting from the rise in plasma fibrinogen and other globulins characteristic of nephrotic syndrome (Chapter 3).

The patient received twice daily infusions of salt-poor albumin followed by intravenous furosemide. With this regimen, blood pressure gradually rose to 100/60 mm Hg and a 5-lb weight loss ensued during the first two hospital days. However, the serum albumin concentration did not rise beyond

ADMISSION LABORATORY DATA, PATIENT 6	
BUN	60 mg/dl
Creatinine	2.0 mg/dl
Albumin	1.1 gm/dl
Erythrocyte Sedimentation Rate	120 mm/hr
Chest X-ray	Large anterior mediastinal mass
Urinalysis	Dipstick: 4+ protein, 0 blood
	Specific gravity: 1.030
	Microscopic examination: Numerous oval fat bodies.

1.3 gm/dl. A 24-hour urine specimen obtained on the second hospital day contained 33.6 gm of protein. Biopsy of the supraclavicular mass on the third hospital day revealed mixed-cellular Hodgkin's disease, clinically Stage IV B.

Systemic chemotherapy was initiated but the patient had a prolonged and stormy hospital course with frequent episodes of hypotension and a bout of *Hemophilus influenzae* pneumonia. He refused renal biopsy. He was discharged two months following admission with objective evidence of tumor regression. Six months later, Hodgkin's disease was in complete remission. At that time, the patient's edema had also resolved and urinalysis was remarkable only for 1+ protein.

Two months later, the patient again developed ankle edema. A chest x-ray revealed a right hilar mass and a large right pleural effusion. Pleural biopsy confirmed recurrent Hodgkin's disease.

Comments: Because intravenously administered albumin is quickly excreted into the urine of nephrotic subjects, albumin infusions are relatively futile in permanently reversing hypoalbuminemia in nephrotic syndrome (see Chapter 6). Considering this patient's profound hypoalbuminemia, heavy proteinuria was not unexpected; however, the reported 24-hour urine protein was measured while he was receiving intravenous albumin and likely overestimated his actual urinary protein excretion.

In this case, the appearance and resolution of heavy proteinuria was temporally correlated with exacerbations and remission of Hodgkin's disease, a pattern that is characteristic of minimal change nephropathy complicating Hodgkin's lymphoma. As discussed in Chapter 4, treatment of nephrotic syndrome associated with malignancies generally consists of therapy for the underlying neoplastic disease. Thus, although renal biopsy was not performed in this case, it seems unlikely that knowledge of the precise glomerular histopathology would have affected the patient's management.

PATIENT 7. A KIDNEY TRANSPLANT RECIPIENT WITH HEAVY PROTEINURIA

A 38-year-old woman developed heavy proteinuria ten months following an otherwise successful cadaveric renal transplantation. Three years earlier, chronic renal failure was discovered when she was evaluated for complaints of anorexia and fatigue. Laboratory studies at that time revealed severe azotemia, proteinuria (3.5 gm per day), and microscopic hematuria with red blood cell casts noted on examination of the urine sediment. Because renal ultrasonography revealed bilaterally atrophic kidneys, biopsy was not performed. The patient was thought to have "chronic glomerulonephritis" and she was prepared for dialysis.

After two years of maintenance hemodialysis, the patient received a cadaveric kidney transplant and had an uncomplicated postoperative course. Immunosuppression was maintained with prednisone and azathioprine. Six months following the transplant, hypertension developed but was well controlled with metolazone and methyldopa. During the subsequent four months, the serum creatinine concentration gradually rose from 1.5 mg/dl to 2.1 mg/dl. A 24-hour urine specimen contained 4.2 gm of protein. Physical examination was unremarkable.

Biopsy of the renal allograft revealed striking glomerular abnormalities with mesangial proliferation and interposition of mesangial matrix between layers of basement membrane resulting in a "tram-track" appearance of the glomerular capillary membrane. Immunofluorescence microscopy revealed subendothelial deposits of C3 and IgG. These pathologic findings suggested membranoproliferative glomerulonephritis.

Comments: Excessive urinary protein excretion is very common in kidney transplant recipients. In fact, heavy proteinuria occurs in as many as 30% of transplant patients. Although chronic allograft rejection is the most common cause of post-transplant nephrotic syndrome, recurrent or de novo glomerular disease must be considered when the transplant recipient develops heavy proteinuria.

Because biopsy of this patient's native kidneys was never performed, one can only speculate whether membranoproliferative changes in the renal allograft represented recurrence of her original glomerular disease. Moreover, the pathologic differentiation of true membranoproliferative disease from the glomerular changes associated with chronic allograft rejection can be difficult. Nevertheless, it has been estimated that as many as 30%→50% of patients with an original diagnosis of membranoproliferative glomerulonephritis develop recurrence of the disease following renal transplantation. Recurrent disease is more common in patients with Type II membranoproliferative glomerulonephritis or "dense-deposit" disease (see Chapter 5).

PATIENT 8. AN ELDERLY WOMAN WITH NEPHROTIC SYNDROME

A 69-year-old woman was hospitalized for evaluation of edema and proteinuria. Past medical history was remarkable for the discovery of glucose intolerance five years earlier. Hyperglycemia was subsequently controlled by diet and weight reduction. The patient also complained of low back pain of more than two years duration. One month prior to admission, the patient noted symmetrical ankle edema. Evaluation at that time included a 24-hour urine collection which revealed 5.2 gm of protein. Dietary sodium restriction was prescribed but the patient's edema progressively worsened. The patient was taking no medications.

On physical examination, blood pressure was 128/85 mm Hg. Fundoscopic examination was normal. A firm 2 × 3-cm mass was palpable in the left upper quadrant of the left breast, but no axillary lymphadenopathy was appreci-

ADMISSION LABORATORY DATA, PATIENT 8	
BUN	16 mg/dl
Creatinine	1.1 mg/dl
Fasting blood sugar	110 mg/dl
Albumin	2.1 gm/dl
ANA	Negative
C3, C4	Normal
Cholesterol	300 mg/dl
Triglyceride	180 mg/dl
Urinalysis	Dipstick: 4+ protein, trace blood, 0 glucose, 0 ketones Microscopic: rare droplets with Maltese-cross pattern viewed under polarized light
24-hour urine protein	5.4 gm
Chest x-ray	Normal
Lumbosacral spine x-ray	Generalized osteopenia; compression fracture of L4.

ated. There was 2+ pitting edema of the ankles to the level of the knees. Neurological examination revealed no motor or sensory deficits. Rectal and pelvic examinations were normal and a stool specimen was guaiac-negative.

Comments: This patient exhibited all of the classic features of nephrotic syndrome. As discussed in Chapter 6, the first task of the physician in such a case is to determine whether the patient has primary or secondary nephrotic syndrome. Considering this patient's history of glucose intolerance, diabetic nephropathy merits some consideration but is exceedingly unlikely in view of the relatively short history of hyperglycemia and the absence of diabetic retinopathy or neuropathy (see Chapter 4). The medical history suggests no drugs or toxins that can be implicated as the cause of proteinuria. Serological studies exclude systemic lupus erythematosus. The patient's breast mass is worrisome because breast cancer is one of a number of malignancies that have been associated with nephrotic syndrome (see Chapter 4). Multiple myeloma and secondary amyloidosis warrant serious consideration in this elderly woman with chronic low back pain, generalized osteopenia, and a lumbar compression fracture.

Bilateral mammograms were remarkable only for changes compatible with fibrocystic disease. An excisional biopsy of the left breast mass revealed a benign adenoma. Serum immunoelectrophoresis showed no monoclonal spike. Urine immunoelectrophoresis did not reveal Bence-Jones proteins. Congo red stain of a subcutaneous fat pad aspirate was negative. Percutaneous renal biopsy was performed. Light microscopic examination revealed diffuse thickening of the glomerular basement membrane. Immunofluorescence microscopy demonstrated deposits of IgG and C3 along the glomerular capillary membrane. Electron microscopy revealed numerous electron-dense subepithelial deposits in the subepithelial portion of the basement membrane.

Comments: The renal biopsy findings suggest membranous glomerulopathy. As discussed in Chapter 6, the histologic abnormalities of membranous glomerulopathy are common to a number of secondary forms of nephrotic syndrome. Thus, the ultimate diagnosis of idiopathic nephrotic syndrome in this case could be made only after the common forms of secondary nephrotic syndrome were excluded on clinical grounds.

The patient received prednisone, 120 mg q.o.d. for two months and experienced no adverse side effects from steroid therapy. After completing two months of treatment, 24-hour urinary protein excretion was 5.8 gm; the serum creatinine concentration was 1.2 mg/dl. Prednisone was gradually tapered and discontinued.

Comments: The treatment of idiopathic membranous glomerulopathy remains a subject of controversy (see Chapter 5). In most patients with this disorder, renal failure develops only after several years of persistent proteinuria. Thus, many nephrologists would have opted to withhold steroid therapy from this elderly woman—especially since prednisone may exacerbate underlying senile osteoporosis. On the other hand, results of the Collaborative Study of Nephrotic Syndrome suggest that a two-month course of alternate day high-dose prednisone therapy exerts a protective influence against the development of renal failure in idiopathic membranous glomerulopathy. Because proteinuria persisted following two months of prednisone, this patient's long-term renal prognosis remains guarded.

Index

A

Acetic acid and heat method, 13–14
Acidosis: renal tubular, 58
Aged: nephrotic syndrome, 186–188
Albumin
    catabolism of, 19, 47
    concentration, and mastectomy, 104
    synthesis, hepatic, 46
    tubular reabsorption of, 19
Amyloidosis, 71, 90–95
    albuminuria and, 104–105
    classification, 92
    clinical features, 93–94
    dialysis and, 95
    epidemiology, 90–91
    pathology, 91
    pathophysiology, 91–93
    proteinuria and Hodgkin's disease, 102
    reactive, 93
    renal biopsy in, 94
    secondary, 93
    systemic, renal histology in, 92
    transplantation and, 95
    treatment, 94–95
Analbuminemia: congenital, 50
Anemia: iron deficiency, 55
Antiglomerular basement membrane disease, 33
Antihypertensive treatment: in diabetic nephropathy, 79
Anti-inflammatory agents, nonsteroidal, 61
    in edema, 161–163
    in hypoalbuminemia, 161–163
    nephrotic syndrome and, 97–98
    renal failure and, acute, 163
Arthritis: rheumatoid, with heavy proteinuria, 182–184
Assays
    quantitative, for urine protein, 5–7
    semiquantitative, for proteinuria, 3
Atherosclerosis: accelerated, 57

B

Bacterial endocarditis, 107–108
Basement membrane
    antiglomerular basement membrane disease, 33
    depositis, location in immune-complex glomerulonephritis, 35
Bence-Jones protein, 5
    myeloma cells and, 92
Biopsy, kidney
    in amyloidosis, 94
    avoided during pregnancy, 110
    in glomerulopathy, idiopathic membranous, 122
    in glomerulosclerosis
        diabetic, 71
        focal segmental, 134
    in lupus nephritis, 86

Biopsy, kidney *(cont.)*
  in minimal change disease, electron micrograph of specimen, 128
  in nephrotic syndrome, 155
    idiopathic, 155–157
  in poststreptococcal glomerulonephritis, acute, 106
  in proteinuria
    asymptomatic, persistent, 152
    heavy, 155

C

Cancer, 101–105
  glomerular pathology associated with, 102
  in glomerulopathy, membranous, 124
Captopril: proteinuria after, 98
Carcinoma, 101
  glomerulopathy and, membranous, 102
Cases, 175–188
Cell-mediated
  immune mechanisms, 33
  mechanisms of glomerular injury, 38–39
Children
  nephropathy, minimal change, 169
  nephrotic syndrome *(see* Nephrotic syndrome, in children)
Complement
  factor B, 59
  in glomerulonephritis, membranoproliferative, 140
  mediating proteinuria, 36–38
  3
    concentration in type II membranoproliferative glomerulonephritis, 141
  nephritic factor, 140
Copper deficiency, 55
Corticosteroids: response in minimal change disease, 131
Creatinine concentration: ratio of urinary protein to, 5
Cyclophosphamide, 89
Cytotoxic drugs: in nephrotic syndrome, in children, 132

D

Dextran: clearance in minimal change nephropathy, 29
Diabetes mellitus, 69–80
  clinical features, 75–77
  epidemiology, 69–70
  glomerulosclerosis of, 30, 71
    renal biopsy in, 71
  nephropathy of *(see* Nephropathy, diabetic)
  pathology, 70–72
  pathophysiology, 72–75
  proteinuria and, asymptomatic persistent, 151–152
  treatment, 78–80
Dialysis, 79
  in amyloidosis, 95
  in glomerulonephritis, membranoproliferative, 143
  in glomerulopathy, membranous, 126
  in lupus erythematosus, systemic, 90
Diet
  in edema, 158–159
  in hypoalbuminemia, 158–159
Dipstick test, 3
Diuresis: in minimal change disease for renal insufficiency, 130
Diuretics, 61
  action sites, 159
  in edema, 159–161
  in hypoalbuminemia, 159–161
Drug(s), 95–101
  anti-inflammatory *(see* Anti-inflammatory agents)
  cytotoxic, in frequently relapsing nephrotic syndrome, in children, 132

E

Edema, 45, 48–51
  anti-inflammatory agents in, nonsteroidal, 161–163
  diet in, 158–159
  diuretics in, 159–161
  management, 158–164
  plasma expanders in, 161
Elderly: nephrotic syndrome in, 186–188
Electron micrograph of biopsy
  in glomerulopathy, idiopathic membranous, 122
  in minimal change disease, 128
Electrophoretic patterns: of abnormal protein excretion, 26
Endocarditis: bacterial, 107–108
Exercise, 39

F

Fanconi syndrome, 27
  full-blown, 58
  tubulointerstitial disease and, 93
Fever, familial Mediterranean, 92, 93
  treatment, 94
Filtration fraction (*see* Glomerulus, filtration fraction)
Flank pain: with gross hematuria, 177–179

G

Glomerular proteinuria (*see* Proteinuria, glomerular)
Glomerular sclerosis (*see* Glomerulosclerosis)
Glomerulonephritis
  focal proliferative, 81
  immune-complex, 33
    basement membrane deposits in, location of, 35
    in situ, 35
  membranoproliferative, 12, 71, 119, 138–143
    clinical features, 141–142
    complement in, 140
    dialysis in, 143
    epidemiology, 138
    lipodystrophy and, 140
    pathology, 138–139
    pathophysiology, 140–141
    therapy, 142–143
    transplant in, 143
    type I, 138, 139
    type II, 138
    type II, C3 concentration in, 141
  membranous, and lupus nephritis, 83
  mesangioproliferative, 143–144
  poststreptococcal, 105–107
    acute, renal biopsy in, 106
Glomerulopathy
  membranoproliferative, and hepatitis B, 108
  membranous, 12, 98, 119–126
    cancer and, 124
    carcinoma and, 102
    clinical features, 124–125
    course in adults, long-term, 125
    dialysis in, 126
    epidemiology, 119
    gold and, 96
    hepatitis B and, 108
    idiopathic, biopsy specimen from, 122
    idiopathic, histologic spectrum of, 121
    idiopathic, penicillamine and, 100
    pathogenesis, 122–124
    pathology, 119–122
    silver stain of glomerulus in, 121
    therapy, 125–126
    thrombosis and, renal vein, 124
    transplant in, 126
  mesangioproliferative, and hepatitis B, 108

Glomerulosclerosis
  diabetic, 30, 71
    renal biopsy in, 71
  focal, 12, 32, 119, 131, 133–138
    clinical features, 136–137
    eipdemiology, 133
    pathogenesis, 135–136
    pathology, 133–135
    segmental, renal biopsy in, 134
    therapy, 137–138
    transplant in, 136
  nodular, 71
    intercapillary, renal tissue in, 72
Glomerulus
  capillary membrane
    tracer proteins in, localization of, 23
    ultrastructure of, 22
  filtration fraction, 39, 50
    influence on urinary protein excretion, 40
  filtration rate after antihypertensive treatment, 79
  histopathology and urinary protein excretion selectivity, 154
  "hyperfiltration," 20, 73
  immune-complex formation, mechanisms of, 32–36
  injury
    cell-mediated mechanisms of, 38–39
    immunologic mechanisms of, 32–39
    mediators of, 38
  pathology associated with neoplasia, 102
  permeability to plasma proteins, increase in, and heavy proteinuria, 48
  properties of
    change-selective, 24–25
    size-selective, 21–23
  sclerosis (see Glomerulosclerosis)
  silver stain in membranous glomerulopathy, 121
Gold, 95–97
  glomerulopathy and, membranous, 96

H

Heart failure, congestive, 39
  nephrotic syndrome and, 175–177
Heat and acetic acid method, 13–14
Hematuria: gross, with flank pain, 177–179
Heparan sulfate, 25
Hepatitis B, 108–109
Heroin, 99–100
  "nephropathy," 99, 134
Hodgkin's disease, 101
  amyloidosis and proteinuria, 102
  minimal change disease and, 128
  with nephrotic syndrome, 184–185
Hypercoagulability mechanisms: in nephrotic syndrome, 62
Hypercoagulable state, 56, 62
Hyperfiltration
  glomerular, 20, 73
  in nephron, 31, 32
Hyperlipidemia, 45, 51–54
  atherosclerosis and proteinuria, 57
  consequences of, 57
  management, 164
  pathogenesis in nephrotic syndrome, 51
Hypoalbuminemia, 45, 46–48
  anti-inflammatory agents in, nonsteroidal, 161–163
  diet in, 158–159
  diuretics in, 159–161
  effects on intrarenal hemodynamics, 162
  lipoprotein metabolism in nephrotic syndrome and, 52
  management, 158–164
  plasma expanders in, 161
  prostaglandin synthesis and, 162
Hypercalcemia, 56

Index

Hypocomplementemia: in SLE, 87
Hypogammaglobulinemia, 55
Hyponatremia, 58–59

I

IgA nephropathy, 144
Immune
  complex(es)
    circulating, size of, 34
    formation, glomerular,
      mechanisms of, 32–36
    formation, in situ, in
      membranous glomerulopathy,
      123–124
    glomerulonephritis (see
      Glomerulonephritis, immune-
      complex)
  mechanisms, cell-mediated, 33
Immunoglobulin A nephropathy, 144
Immunologic mechanisms: of
  glomerular injury, 32–39
Immunologically induced
  proteinuria: inflammatory
  mediators of, 36–38
Infection complicating heavy
  proteinuria, 59–60
  management, 166–167
Infectious diseases: and nephrotic
  syndrome, 105–109
Intrarenal hemodynamic factors: in
  proteinuria, 31–32
Iron deficiency
  anemia, 55
  management, 165

K

Kidney
  biopsy (see Biopsy, kidney)
  disease
    nonglomerular, proteinuria
      mechanisms in, 31–32
    protein excretion patterns in,
      26–28
    proteinuria absent in, 2
    proteinuria as first sign of, 1
    proteinuria in, mechanisms of,
      25–30
  failure
    acute, complicating heavy
      proteinuria, 60–61
    anti-inflammatory agents and,
      nonsteroidal, 163
    hemodynamics, effects of heavy
      proteinuria and
      hypoalbuminemia on, 162
  histology
    in amyloidosis, systemic, 92
    resembling nephrotic syndrome,
      idiopathic, 156
  insufficiency in minimal change
    disease, 130
  intrarenal hemodynamic factors in
    proteinuria, 31–32
  in Kimmelstiel Wilson disease, 72
  normal, protein-handling by,
    17–25
  plasma flow after antihypertensive
    treatment, 79
  transplant (see Transplantation,
    kidney)
  tubule
    acidosis, 58
    dysfunction, proximal, 57–58
    proteinuria, protein excretion
      pattern in, 27
    reabsorption of albumin, 19
  vein thrombosis (see Thrombosis,
    renal vein)
Kimmelstiel Wilson disease, 71
  renal tissue in, 72

L

Lipiduria, 8, 45, 51–54
Lipodystrophy, 138
  glomerulonephritis and,
    membranoproliferative, 140
Lipoprotein metabolism: in
  nephrotic syndrome, and
  hypoalbuminemia, 52

Liver: albumin synthesis, 46
Lupus
  erythematosus, systemic, 80–90
    clinical features, 84–87
    dialysis and, 90
    epidemiology, 80–81
    pathology, 81–83
    pathophysiology, 83–84
    therapy, 87–90
    transplantation and, 90
  nephritis, 80
    chronicity index, 86
    clinical features, 84
    diffuse proliferative, 81, 82–83
    focal proliferative, 81
    histologic patterns, four basic, 82
    management, treatment strategy, 88
    membranous, 81
    mesangial, 81
    renal biposy in, 86
Lymphocytes, 38
Lysozymuria, 28

M

Macroglobulinemia: Waldenstrom's, 105
Macrophages, 39
Malnutrition, 59
Mastectomy: protein excretion and albumin concentration, 104
MCD (see Minimal change disease)
Mediterranean fever, familial, 92, 93
  treatment, 94
Metabolic abnormalities: associated with nephrotic syndrome, 157–164
Microalbuminuria, 73
Minimal change disease, 102, 119, 127–133
  biopsy specimen from, electron micrograph of, 128
  clinical features, 129–130
  corticosteroids in, response to, 131
  epidemiology, 127
  Hodgkin's disease and, 128
  pathogenesis, 127–129
  pathology, 127
  renal insufficiency in, reversal in response to diuresis, 130
  therapy, 130–133
Minimal change nephropathy (see Nephropathy, minimal change)
Myeloma
  cells, and Bence Jones proteins, 92
  multiple, 5, 90, 101
    nephrotic syndrome complicating, 104
    proteinuria pattern in, 27

N

Neoplasia (see Cancer)
Nephrectomy: in proteinuria, 164
Nephritic factor: C3, 140
Nephritis
  glomerulonephritis (see Glomerulonephritis)
  lupus (see Lupus, nephritis)
Nephron: hyperfiltration in, 31, 32
Nephropathy
  diabetic, 69
    antihypertensive treatment, 79
    management, 78–80
    pathogenesis of, postulated mechanisms, 74
    type I, clinical course, 76
  "heroin," 99, 134
  IgA, 144
  light chain, 71
    discussion of, 105
  minimal change, 29
    in children, 169
    dextran clearance in, 29
Nephrotic syndrome
  in aged, 186–188
  assessment, clinical and laboratory, 152–155
  biopsy in, renal, 155

in children, 149
  distribution by histopathology, 170
  frequently relapsing nephrotic syndrome, 179–180
  frequently relapsing nephrotic syndrome, cytotoxic drugs in, 132
  management, 169–171
  steroids in, response prediction, 171
complicating multiple myeloma, 104
consequences of heavy proteinuria, 45–67
definition of, 45
drugs associated with, 96
etiology, 64
frequently relapsing, in children, 179–180
  cytotoxic drugs in, 132
with heart failure, congestive, 175–177
heroin and, 99–100
with Hodgkin's disease, 184–185
hypercoagulability in, mechanisms of, 62
hyperlipidemia pathogenesis in, 51
idiopathic, 119–148
  adult, clinical features, 120
  biopsy in, renal, 155–157
  disorders in which renal histopathology resembles, 156
  lipoprotein metabolism in, and hypoalbuminemia, 52
  management, 152–155
  metabolic abnormalities associated with, 157–164
  pregnancy complicating, 109–110
  protein deficiencies in, serum, 56
  protein electrophoreses in, serum, 55
  proteinuria and, asymptomatic, 11
secondary
  amyloidosis and, 90–95
  anti-inflammatory drugs and, nonsteroidal, 97–98
  assessment, 153
  causes of, 70
  diabetes and, 69–80
  disorders associated with, 69–117
  drugs and, 95–101
  infectious diseases and, 105–109
  lupus erythematosus and, systemic, 80–90
  toxins and, 95–101
  thromboembolism in, mechanisms of, 62
  urine sediment in, 54
Neutrophils: mediating proteinuria, 36–38

O

Orthostatic proteinuria, 10

P

Pain: flank, with gross hematuria, 177–179
Penicillamine: proteinuria after, 100–101
Plasma
  expanders
    in edema, 161
    in hypoalbuminemia, 161
  volumes, 50
    hyponatremia and, 58
Poststreptococcal glomerulonephritis, 105–107
  acute, renal biopsy in, 106
Postural proteinuria, 10
Prednisone, 89
Preeclampsia, 109
Pregnancy
  nephrotic syndrome complicating, 109–110
  renal biopsy avoided during, 110
Prostaglandin synthesis
  hypoalbuminemia and, 162

Prostaglandin synthesis *(cont.)*
  proteinuria and, heavy, 162
Protein
  Bence-Jones, 5
    myeloma cells and, 92
  excretion
    abnormal, electrophoretic
      patterns of, 26
    in kidney disease, patterns of,
      26–28
  -handling by normal kidney,
    17–25
  plasma
    binding deficiencies,
      management, 165–166
    glomerular permeability
      increase to, 48
  precipitation techniques, 3
  serum
    abnormalities of, 54–56
    deficiencies in nephrotic
      syndrome, 56
    electrophoreses in nephrotic
      syndrome, 55
  tracer, localization in glomerular
    capillary membrane, 23
  urine
    excretion, and glomerular
      histopathology, 154
    excretion, influence of filtration
      fraction on, 40
    excretion, mastectomy and, 104
    excretion, theoretical
      mechanisms of, 18
    positive test for, approach to
      "healthy" patient with, 7
    quantitative assays for, 5–7
    ratio to creatinine
      concentration, 5
Proteinuria
  absence in kidney disease, 2
  asymptomatic, 11, 149
  -assessment, 150–152
    evaluation, follow-up, 150
    management, 150–152
    persistent, assessment, 151–152
    persistent, biopsy in, 152
    persistent, diabetes and,
      151–152
    persistent, management,
      151–152
  benign transient, 7, 8–9
    assessment, 150
    management, 150
  after captopril, 98
  classification of, 1–15
    table, 9
  complement mediating, 36–38
  detection of, 1–15
    methods, 2–7
    semiquantitative precipitation
      tests for, 13
  diagnosis, 149–174
  at first sign of kidney disease, 1
  functional, 9
    assessment, 150–151
    causes, common, 10
    management, 150–151
    mechanisms of, 39–40
  glomerular
    molecular basis of, 28–30
    "nonselective" pattern, 26
    protein excretion patterns in, 26
    "selective" pattern, 26
  heavy, 11
    assessment, 152–155
    complications of, life-
      threatening, 59–65
    consequences of, 45–67
    consequences of, common, 46–54
    consequences from increased
      glomerular permeability to
      plasma proteins, 48
    consequences of, management
      of, 165–169
    consequences of, miscellaneous,
      54–59
    effects on intrarenal
      hemodynamics, 162
    infection complicating, 59–60
    infection complicating,
      management, 166–167

kidney failure complicating,
    acute, 60–61
after kidney transplant,
    185–186
management, 152–155
prostaglandin synthesis and,
    162
renal biopsy in, 155
with rheumatoid arthritis,
    182–184
thromboembolism complicating,
    61–65
vascular collapse complicating,
    60–61
Hodgkin's disease and
    amyloidosis, 102
hyperlipidemia and
    atherosclerosis, 57
immunologically induced,
    inflammatory mediators,
    36–38
intermittent, 8–11, 149
    assessment, 150–152
    case, illustrative, 181
    evaluation, follow-up, 150
    management, 150–152
management, general, 149–174
mechanisms of, 17–43
    in kidney disease, 25–30
    in kidney disease,
        nonglomerular, 31–32
mediators of, 38
nephrectomy in, 164
neutrophils mediating, 36–38
orthostatic, 10
"overflow," 20
overproduction, 27–28
after penicillamine, 100–101
persistent, 11–13
postural, 10, 150
    assessment, 151
    biopsy in, 151
    management, 151
quantitation methods, 2–7
semiquantitative assays for, 3
    false-negative, 5

false-positive, 3–4
false-positive, causes of, 4
tubular, protein excretion pattern
    in, 27
Proteinuric states
    classification of, 1–15
    table, 9
    detection, 1–15

R

Renal
    (*See also* Kidney)
    vein thrombosis (*see* Thrombosis,
        renal vein)
Rheumatoid arthritis: with heavy
    proteinuria, 182–184

S

Sclerosis, glomerular (*see*
    Glomerulosclerosis)
Serum sickness, 34
Steroids: in nephrotic syndrome,
    response prediction in
    children, 171
Sulfosalicylic acid
    method, 13
    turbidity test, quantitative, 14

T

Thromboembolism
    mechanisms in nephrotic
        syndrome, 62
    proteinuria complicated by. heavy,
        61–65
Thrombosis, renal vein, 60, 61
    in glomerulopathy, membranous,
        124
    incidence, 64
    management, 167–169
Toxins, 95–101
Transferrin deficiency, 55
Transplantation, kidney, 79
    in amyloidosis, 95

Transplantation, kidney *(cont.)*
  in glomerulonephritis,
    membranoproliferative, 143
  in glomerulopathy, membranous,
    126
  in glomerulosclerosis, gocal, 136
  in lupus erythematosus, systemic,
    90
  in proteinuria, heavy, 185–186
Tubule (*see* Kidney, tubule)
Tubulointerstitial diseases, 31
Tumors (*see* Cancer)

U

Ultrastructure: of glomerular
  capillary membrane, 22

Urine
  protein (*see* Protein, urine)
  sediment in nephrotic syndrome,
    54

V

Vascular collapse: complicating
  heavy proteinuria, 60–61
Vein, renal (*see* Thrombosis, renal
  vein)

W

Waldenstrom's macroglobulinemia,
  105